STATISTICS:
A Guide to the Biological and Health Sciences

HOLDEN-DAY SERIES IN PROBABILITY AND STATISTICS

E. L. Lehmann, Editor

Bickel and Doksum: *Mathematical Statistics*
Carlson: *Statistics*
Freedman: *Markov Processes*
Freedman: *Approximating Countable Markov Chains*
Freedman: *Brownian Motion and Diffusion*
Hájek: *Nonparametric Statistics*
Hodges and Lehmann: *Elements of Finite Probability, 2d ed.*
Hodges and Lehmann: *Basic Concepts of Probability and Statistics, 2d ed.*
Lehmann: *Nonparametrics: Statistical Methods Based on Ranks*
Nemenyi, Dixon, White: *Statistics From Scratch*
Neveu: *Mathematical Foundations of the Calculus of Probability*
Parzen: *Stochastic Processes*
Rényi: *Foundations of Probability*
*Roberts: *Interactive Data Analysis*
Tanur, Mosteller, Kruskal, et al: *Statistics: A Guide to the Unknown*
Tanur, Mosteller, Kruskal, et al: *Statistics: A Guide to Business and Economics*
Tanur, Mosteller, Kruskal, et al: *Statistics: A Guide to Biological and Health Sciences*
Tanur, Mosteller, Kruskal, et al: *Statistics: A Guide to Political and Social Issues*
*Waller: *Statistics: An Introduction to Numerical Reasoning*

*To be published

STATISTICS: A Guide to the Biological and Health Sciences

by the editors of
STATISTICS: A GUIDE TO THE UNKNOWN

JUDITH M. TANUR
State University of New York, Stony Brook

and

FREDERICK MOSTELLER, Chairman
Harvard University

WILLIAM H. KRUSKAL
University of Chicago

RICHARD F. LINK
Artronic Information Systems, Inc.

RICHARD S. PIETERS
Phillips Academy, Andover, Mass.

GERALD R. RISING
State University of New York, Buffalo

The Joint Committee on
The Curriculum in Statistics and Probability of
The American Statistical Association and
The National Council of Teachers of Mathematics

and by

E. L. LEHMANN
University of California, Berkeley
Special Editor

 HOLDEN-DAY, INC.
SAN FRANCISCO   London   Dusseldorf   Johannesburg
Panama   Singapore   Sydney

PREFACE

WARREN WEAVER, a great expositor of science, discussed why science is not more widely appreciated and issued a call in "The Imperfections of Science" (*American Scientist*, 49:113, March 1961):

> What we must do—scientists and non-scientists alike—is close the gap. We must bring science back into life as a human enterprise, an enterprise that has at its core the uncertainty, the flexibility, the subjectivity, the sweet unreasonableness, the dependence upon creativity and faith which permit it, when properly understood, to take its place as a friendly and understanding companion to all the rest of life.

As this book makes clear, scientific thinking, most particularly related to statistics, is not restricted to "pure" science, but has many uses in applied fields such as health sciences as well. And most especially, it is necessary to develop what we might call a statistical attitude toward, and manner of thinking about, these disciplines.

To prepare a volume describing important applications of statistics and probability in many fields of endeavor—this was the project that the ASA-NCTM Committee initiated early in 1969 as an effort to close the gap Weaver and others had pointed out. *Statistics: A Guide to the Unknown* (SAGTU) was the result.

During the book's preparation several of us who were working on it and teaching simultaneously found much of the material very useful— even inspirational—to undergraduate and graduate students. It seemed that the book had an additional possible function as an auxiliary textbook. This impression has been confirmed over the years since publication of *SAGTU* as college after college, university after university, and even secondary after secondary school adopted *SAGTU* as an auxiliary textbook for introductory statistics classes.

Instructors and students have reported success in using *SAGTU* as a means of tying techniques and methods, taught necessarily at a simple level with simplified examples, to real problems in the real world. In specialized courses, some teachers wanted sets of essays oriented to their subject matter. Students studying biologic sciences, for example, found themselves only distantly concerned with statistical applications in business and economics. The very diversity of applications that had fascinated us became an impediment to the usefulness of *SAGTU* as an auxiliary textbook within the time constraints of a specialized statistics course. It is for this reason that the decision was taken to compile what we have come to refer to as mini-*SAGTU*'s: each a selection of articles from *SAGTU* (and in this volume, one new article) dealing with a particular field of application—*Statistics: A Guide to the Biological and Health Sciences* (SAGBAHS) is the second such volume to appear. (The first was *Statistics: A Guide to Business & Economics.*)

The essays here, and in *SAGTU* itself, do not teach technical methods, but rather illustrate past accomplishments and current uses of statistics and probability. In choosing the actual essays to include, the Committee aimed at illustrating a variety of applications, but did not attempt the impossible task of covering all possible uses. Even in the areas included, attempts at complete coverage have been deliberately avoided. We discouraged authors from writing essays that could be entitled "All Uses of Statistics in . . . " Rather, we asked authors to stress one or a very few important problems within their field of application and to explain how statistics and probability help to solve them and why the solutions are useful to the nation, to science, or to the people who originally posed the problem. In the past, for those who were unable to cope with very technical material, such essays have been hard to find.

When describing work in the mathematical sciences, one must make a major decision as to what level of mathematics to ask of the reader. Although the Joint Committee serves professional organizations whose subject matter is strongly mathematical, we decided to explain statistical ideas and contributions without dwelling on their mathematical aspects. This was a bold stroke, and our authors were surprised that we largely held firm.

There is an old saw that a camel is a horse put together by a committee. Our authors supplied exceedingly well-formed and attractive anatomical parts, but to the extent that this book gaits well, credit is due primarily to a most talented and dedicated Committee. In general, the approach to unanimity in the Committee's critical reviews of and suggestions about essays was phenomenal. And, though they may have occasionally been divided about the strong and weak points of a particular essay, they were constantly united in their purpose of producing a useful book, and in their ability to find something more than 24 hours a day to work on it. This dedication undoubtedly created difficulties for our authors. Nevertheless, our authors persevered and deserve enormous thanks from us, and from the Committee, and from the statistical profession at large.

Our thanks go also to the Sloan Foundation whose grant made it possible to put this book together.

There are others to thank as well: to the office of the American Statistical Association (and, in particular, to Edgar Bisgyer, and John Lehman, and later Fred Leone) for invaluable help in all the administrative work necessary to get out a book such as this; and similar thanks to the administration of the National Council of Teachers of Mathematics; to Edward Millman for careful and imaginative editorial assistance; and to other people at Holden-Day, especially Frederick H. Murphy, and Erich Lehmann, our Series Editor; to Mrs. Holly Grano for acting as a long-distance and long-haul secretary; and to the many friends and colleagues both of the Editor and of the Committee members who so often acted as unsung, but indispensable, advisors.

In this new effort to compile *SAGBAHS*, additional thanks go to the original Committee members and to the guiding spirit of Erich Lehmann. We also have additional thanks for John Gilbert, Bucknam McPeek, and Frederick Mosteller, the authors of the one new article appearing in this volume, "How frequently do innovations succeed in surgery and anesthesia?" The supplementary material for study, prepared especially for *SAGBAHS* is the valuable contribution of Haiganoush Preisler and Esther Sid.

Frederick Mosteller
Judith Tanur

March, 1977

CONTENTS

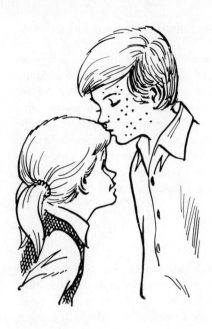

EPIDEMICS

Maurice S. Bartlett   *Oxford University*

[*Editorial comment.* Many advisors have suggested that this volume include an application in which a statistical or stochastic model is especially constructed to fit a real world process. These advisors want the volume to show the reader the model builder at work, to show how the model is tested, and to explore the new things it demonstrates. To appreciate the whole process requires some mathematics. We also might have to see the worker's wastebasket to appreciate how much effort may go into attempts he found unsatisfying.

Even the reader who has little mathematical equipment can gain considerable insight into the mathematical study of the birth, death, and maintenance of epidemics by skipping the harder mathematics in the piece Professor Bartlett has so kindly provided. For those who wish to skip along, the more mathematical parts have been set off and indented, and a few words, sometimes redundant, of transition have been inserted.—J.T.]

A CLASSIC book by the late Professor Greenwood, a medical statistician who was an authority on epidemics, has the title *Epidemics and Crowd Diseases,* which emphasizes the relevance of the population, or community, in determining how epidemics arise and recur. One of the first to realize the need for more than purely empirical studies of epidemic phenomena was Ronald Ross, better known for his discovery of the role of the mosquito in transmitting malaria to human beings. Since those early years, the mechanism and behavior of epidemics arising from infection that spreads from individual to individual, either directly or by an intermediate carrier, have been extensively studied,[1] but it is perhaps fair to say that only in recent years have some quantitative features become understood and even now much remains to be unraveled.

MATHEMATICAL MODELS AND DATA

The statistical study of epidemics, then, has two aspects—on one hand, the medical statistics on some infectious disease of interest and, on the other hand, an appraisal of the theoretical consequences of the mathematical model believed to be representative, possibly in a very simplified and idealized fashion, of the actual epidemic situation. If the consequences of the model seem to agree broadly with the observed characteristics, there is some justification for thinking that the model is on the right lines, especially if it predicts some features that had been unknown, or at least had not been used, when the model was formulated.

How do we build a mathematical model of a population under attack by an infectious agent? There is no golden rule for success. Some feel that everything that is known about the true epidemic situation should be set down and incorporated into the model. Unfortunately, this procedure is liable to provide a very indigestible hotchpotch with which no mathematician can cope, and while in these days of large-scale computers there is much more scope for studying the properties of these possibly realistic, but certainly complicated, models, there is still much to be said for keeping our model as simple as is feasible without too gross a departure from the real state of affairs. Let us begin then at the other extreme and put in our ingredients one at a time.

We start with a community of individuals susceptible to the infection, let us say a number S of them. We must also have some infection, and we will confine our attention to the situation in which this can be represented by a number of individuals already infected and liable to pass on the disease. The astute reader will notice that even if we are concentrating on epidemic situations with person-to-person infection, we perhaps ought not to amalgamate *infected* and *infective* persons. Some people may be already infected, but

---

[1] Other pioneering workers in this field include W. Hamer, A. G. McKendrick, H. E. Soper, and E. B. Wilson.

not yet infective; some might not be infected, at least visibly, and yet be infective—so-called *carriers*. As we are considering the simplest case, however, we merely suppose there is a number I, say, of infective persons. When, as is to be hoped in real life, these persons recover, they may become resusceptible sooner or later (as for the common cold) or permanently immune, as is observed with a very high proportion of people in the case of measles.

While these ingredients for our epidemic recipe are very basic and common to many situations, there is a better check on our model if we are more definite and have one disease in mind, so let us consider only measles from now on. This is largely a children's complaint, mainly because most adults in contact with the virus responsible have already become immune and so do not concern us. Measles is no longer as serious an illness as it used to be (even less now that there is a preventive vaccine), but is a convenient one to discuss because many of its characteristics are fairly definite: the permanence of subsequent immunity, the incubation period of about a fortnight, and the requirement of notifiability in several countries, including the U.S., England, and Wales. The last requirement ensures the existence of official statistics, though it is known that notifications, unfortunately, are far from complete. Provided we bear this last point in mind, however, and where necessary make allowance for incomplete notification, it should not mislead us.

A DETERMINISTIC MATHEMATICAL MODEL

To return to our mock epidemic, we next suppose that the infective persons begin to infect the susceptibles. If the infectives remain infective, all the susceptibles come down with the infection eventually, and that is more or less all there is to be said. A more interesting situation arises when the infective persons may recover (or die, or be removed from contact with susceptibles) because then a competition between the number of new infections of susceptibles and the number of recoveries of infectives is set up. At the beginning of the epidemic, when there may be a large number of susceptibles to be infected, a kind of chain reaction can occur, and the number of notifications of new infected persons may begin to rise rapidly; later on, when there are fewer susceptibles, the rate of new notifications will begin to go down, and the epidemic will subside.

If we drew a graph of the number of infectives I against the number of susceptibles S at each moment, it would look broadly like the curve in Figure 1. The precise path, of course, will depend on the exact assumptions made on the overall rate of infection, on whether this is strictly proportional to the number I, and on whether also proportional to S, so that the rate at any moment is, say, calculated from the formula aIS where a is a constant. The path will depend also on the rate of recovery of the infected population,

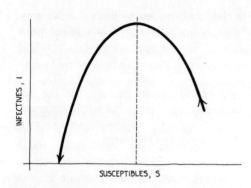

FIGURE 1

General path of an epidemic beginning with many susceptibles S, increasing at first the number of infectives I, then decreasing

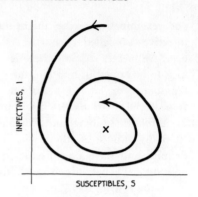

FIGURE 2

Deterministic model. Approach to equilibrium point (at cross) of I, S curve

likely to be proportional to I and given by bI, say, where b is a constant. Without going into too much detail yet, we can note one or two distinct features in the figure: (1) the susceptible population may not be reduced to zero at the time that the sources of infection have been eliminated; (2) because the path has no "memory," we could start at any point on it and proceed along the same curve—if our starting point were to the right of the maximum point, our infectives I would rise, if to the left, they would fall.

Actually, our more detailed assumptions are equivalent to the pair of recurrence relations for calculating I_{t+1}, S_{t+1} at any time $t + 1$ in terms of the values I_t, S_t at the previous time t (the unit of time should be small, say, a day or week):

$$S_{t+1} = S_t - aI_tS_t, \qquad I_{t+1} = I_t + aI_tS_t - bI_t.$$

We notice that $I_{t+1} - I_t$ is positive or negative according to whether $aS_t - b$ is positive or negative. The value b/a for S (on our assumptions it is independent of I) is called the *critical threshold* for reasons that will become clear.

Thus far we have a model for a "closed epidemic," which terminates when I is zero. Can we turn it into a model for measles, which has been claimed to come in epidemics about every two years? One ingredient still missing is an influx of susceptibles, due, in the case of childhood illnesses, to births within the community.

Let us, therefore, add a term c, say, to the right-hand side of the first equation above. If we follow the course of events in Figure 1, the path will start turning right before it reaches the axis $I = 0$ and can be shown to proceed in an ever-decreasing spiral (Figure 2) till it finally arrives at an equilibrium point, which is determined by the equations

$$c - aIS = 0, \qquad aIS - bI = 0.$$

The second of these gives $S = b/a$ (the critical threshold value), and the first then yields $I = c/b$. These results are partly encouraging, but partly erroneous. The encouraging feature is the tendency to recurrent epidemics; we can even find the period of the cycle, which is found to be approximately

$$\frac{2\pi}{\sqrt{ac - \frac{1}{4}a^2c^2/b}}.$$

Sir William Hamer, who first put forward the above model for measles in 1906, took $b = \frac{1}{2}$ when t is reckoned in weeks, corresponding to an average incubation period of a fortnight, and c for London at that time as 2200. The value of a is more uncertain, but one method of arriving at it is to note that the *average* number of susceptibles, which was put at 150,000, should be around the theoretical equilibrium value b/a giving $a = 1/300,000$. Notice that c will tend to be proportional to the size of the community, so that if ac is to remain constant, a must be inversely proportional to the population, but this is not an unreasonable assumption; it is consistent, for example, with effective infectivity over a constant urban area, the entire town being regarded as an assemblage of such units.

The introduction of an influx of susceptibles showed that instead of following the simple curved path of Figure 1, an epidemic might follow a spiral until it finally settled down with a particular number of susceptibles. The time to go around the spiral once, called the *period*, is estimated for London data at 74 weeks, in reasonable agreement with the average period of somewhat less than two years that has been observed for large towns in England and Wales (see Table 2), the U.S. and comparable countries in the present century. We would hardly expect the epidemic pattern to remain precisely the same under very different social conditions, though the annual measles mortality figures for London quoted from John Graunt for the seventeenth century (Table 1) suggest a similar pattern even then (with perhaps a slightly longer average period of 2 to 3 years).

TABLE 1. Deaths from Measles in London in the Seventeenth Century

1629	1630	1631	1632	1633	1634	1635	1636	1637–46	1647	1648
41	2	3	80	21	33	27	12	Not recorded	5	92

1649	1650	1651	1652	1653	1654	1655	1656	1657	1658	1659	1660
3	33	33	62	8	52	11	153	15	80	6	74

UNSATISFACTORY FEATURES OF THE MODEL

The erroneous feature of the improved model is that actual measles in London or other large towns recurs in epidemics without settling down to a steady endemic state represented by the theoretical equilibrium point. What aspects of our model must we correct? There are some obvious points to look at:

(1) Our assumptions about the rate of recovery correspond to a gradual and steadily decreasing fraction of any group infected at the same time, whereas the incubation period is fairly precise at about two weeks, before the rash appears and the sick child is likely to be isolated (this being equivalent to recovery).

(2) We have ignored the way the children are distributed over the town, coming to school if they are old enough or staying at home during a vacation period.

(3) Measles is partly seasonal in its appearance, with a swing in average notifications from about 60% below average in summer to 60% above average in winter.

INTRODUCING CHANCE INTO THE MODEL

We will consider these points in turn. The effect of point (1) is to lessen the "damping down" to the equilibrium level, but not, when correctly formulated, to eliminate it. Point (2), on the movement over the town, raises interesting questions about the rate of spread of infection across different districts, but is less relevant to the epidemic pattern in time, except for its possible effect on (3). If we postulate a ±10% variation in the "coefficient of infectivity" a over the year, it is found to account for the observed ±60% or so in notifications. There seems to be little evidence of an intrinsic change in a due, say, to weather conditions, and it may well be an artifact arising from dispersal for the long summer vacation and crowding together of children after the holidays. Whatever its cause, it does not explain the persistence of a natural period; only the seasonal variation would remain and give a strict annual period, still at variance with observation.

To proceed further, let us retrace our steps to our closed epidemic model of Figure 1. To fix our ideas, suppose we initially had only one infective individual in the community. Then the course of events is not certain to be as depicted; it may happen that this individual recovers (or is isolated) before passing on the infection, even if the size of susceptible population is above the critical threshold. This emphasizes the chance element in epidemics, especially at the beginning of the outbreak, and this element is specifically introduced by means of probability theory. To examine the difference it makes, let us suppose the *chance* P of a new infection is now proportional to aIS and the chance Q of a recovery proportional to bI. Denote the chance of the outbreak ultimately fading out without causing a major epidemic by p. We shall suppose also that the initial number S_0 of susceptibles is large enough for us not to worry about the proportionate change in S if the (small) number of infective persons changes. Under these conditions two infective persons can be thought of as acting independently in spreading infection, so that the chance of the outbreak fading out with *two* initial infective persons must be p^2.

Now consider the situation after the first "happening." Either this is a new infection or a recovery, and the relative odds are $P/Q = aS_0/b$. If it is a new infection, I changes from 1 to 2, and the chance of fade-out is p^2 from now on, or I drops to zero, and fade-out has already occurred. This gives the relation

$$p = \frac{P}{P+Q}p^2 + \frac{Q}{P+Q},$$

whence either $p = 1$ or $p = Q/P = b/(aS_0)$. If $b \geq aS_0$ (that is, if we are below the critical threshold) the only possible solution is $p = 1$, implying as expected that the outbreak certainly fades out. However, the ultimate probability of fade-out can be envisaged as the final value reached by the probability of fade-out up to some definite time t, this more general probability steadily increasing from zero at $t = 0$ to its limiting value, which therefore will be the *smaller* of the roots of the above quadratic equation. This is $b/(aS_0)$ if this value is less than one, providing us with a quantitative (nonzero) value of the chance of fade-out *even if the critical threshold is exceeded* and stressing the new and rather remarkable complications that arise when probabilistic concepts are brought in.

The mathematics shows that if the initial number of susceptibles is smaller than a value determined by the ratio of some rates used in the model, then the epidemic will certainly fade out. If it is larger than this critical value, then there is still a positive probability that the epidemic will fade out.

When new susceptibles are continually introduced, represented by c, the complications are even greater. For small communities, however, the qualitative features can be guessed. Once below the threshold, the number of infectives will tend to drop to zero, and though the susceptibles S can increase because of c, it seems unlikely that the number will pass the threshold before I has dropped to zero. The epidemic is now finished, and cannot re-start unless we introduce some *new* infection from outside the community. This is exactly what is observed with measles in a small isolated community, whether it is a boarding school, a rural village, or an island community. For such communities, the period between epidemics depends partly on the rate of immigration of new infection into the area and not just on the natural epidemic cycle. Moreover, when new infection enters, it cannot take proper hold if the susceptible population is still below the threshold, and even if

TABLE 2.   Measles Epidemics for Towns in England and Wales (1940–56)

TOWN	POPULATION (THOUSANDS)	MEAN PERIOD BETWEEN EPIDEMICS (WEEKS)	TOWN	POPULATION (THOUSANDS)	MEAN PERIOD BETWEEN EPIDEMICS (WEEKS)
Birmingham	1046	73	Newbury	18	92
Manchester	658	106	Carmarthen	12	79
Bristol	415	92	Penrith	11	98
Hull	269	93	Ffestiniog	7.1	199
Plymouth	180	94	Brecon	5.6	149
Norwich	113	80	Okehampton	4.0	105
Barrow-in-Furness	66	74	Cardigan	3.5	>284
Carlisle	65	75	South Molton	3.1	191
Bridgwater	22	86	Llanrwst	2.6	>284
			Appleby	1.7	175

Source: Bartlett (1957), Tables 1 and 2.

above, new infection may have to enter a few times before a major outbreak occurs. The average period tends to be above the natural period for such communities. If we assume that the rate of immigration of new infection is likely to be proportional to the population of the community, the average period between epidemics will tend to be larger the smaller the community, and this again is what is observed (Table 2).

Consider now a larger community. We expect random effects to be proportionately less; there is still, however, the possibility of extinction when the critical threshold is not exceeded. Nevertheless, before all the infectives have disappeared, the influx c of new susceptibles may have swung S above the threshold, and the stage is set for a new epidemic. Under these conditions (and provided ac remains constant, as already assumed), the natural period will change little with the size of community.

CRITICAL SIZE OF COMMUNITY

How large does the community have to be if it is to begin to be independent of outside infection and if its epidemic cycle is to be semipermanent? Exact mathematical results are difficult to obtain, but approximate solutions have been supplemented by simulation studies of the epidemic model, using computers. An example of one such series plotted to extinction of infection after four epidemics (an interval representing nearly seven years) is shown in Figure 3. This particular series has no built-in seasonal incidence, but some internal

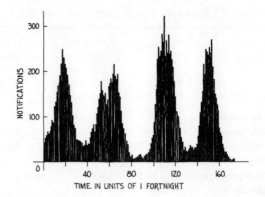

FIGURE 3

Results of simulation of four epidemics of measles over a seven-year period for a town whose average susceptible population is 3700

migration within its population boundaries; its average susceptible population is 3700. It appears from all such results that the critical size of the susceptible population is, for the measles model, of the order of 7000, or if the factor of 40 estimated for Manchester, England, between total and susceptible population is used, over a quarter of a million people in the community.

Now we do not need to use this theoretical figure as more than an indication of what to look for. By direct examination of measles notifications for any town, we can see whether notifications have been absent for more than two or three weeks. In view of the rather well-defined incubation period, we would infer from this lack of notifications that the infection had disappeared if we knew that notifications were complete. Incomplete notification is a complication, but not one that is likely to affect these quantitative conclusions very much, for fade-out of infection is found to increase rather rapidly as the community size decreases and soon becomes quite recognizable from the detailed statistics. In this way, it was ascertained that in England and Wales, during the period 1940–56, cities of critical size were Bristol (population about 415,000) and Hull (269,000). This investigation was supplemented by an examination of U.S. statistics for the period 1921–40, from which it was found that some comparable North American cities were Akron (245,000), Providence (254,000), and Rochester (325,000). Therefore, there is an observed critical community size of around 300,000, in reasonable agreement with what we were expecting.

Of course, towns of such size are not completely isolated from other communities as assumed in our model; this could tend to lessen the observed critical size, especially if the isolation is comparatively slight. In Table 3 the fade-out effect is shown for aggregates of individual "wards" in Manchester to demonstrate how it decreases with the population aggregate. The critical size (defined precisely in terms of 50% probability of fade-out after an epidemic) is, again as expected, smaller than for complete towns due to the

TABLE 3.   Observed (Aggregate) Fade-Out Effect in Manchester Wards

WARDS	CUMULATIVE POPULATION (THOUSANDS)	NUMBER OF EPIDEMICS FOLLOWED BY FADE-OUT	PROBABILITY OF FADE-OUT (%)
Ardwick	18.4	12	100
St. Mark's	38.2	12	100
St. Luke's and New Cross	71.8	9	75
All Saints, Beswick, and Miles Platting	140.8	4	33
Openshaw, Longsight, N. and S. Gorton, Bradford, and St. Michaels	254.1	1	8
Medlock St., W. and E. Moss Side, Rusholme, Newton Heath, Collyhurst, Harpurhey, and Cheetham	419.3	0	0

Source: Bartlett (1957), Table 3.

extensive migration across the ward boundaries; it is estimated to be 120,000 total population living within the area.

CONCLUSIONS

If we review these results, we may justifiably claim that our theoretical model for measles, idealized though it inevitably is, has achieved some fair degree of agreement with the observed epidemic pattern.   In particular:

(1) It predicts a "natural" period between epidemics of rather less than two years.

(2) A small ($\pm 10\%$) seasonal variation in infectivity (whether or not an artifact of seasonal pattern in school-children's movements) accounts for the larger ($\pm 60\%$) observed seasonal variation in notifications.

(3) It predicts extinction of infection for small communities, with consequent extension (and greater variability) of periods between epidemics.

(4) It predicts a critical community size of over a quarter of a million necessary for the infection to remain in the community from one epidemic to the next.

Epidemic patterns, of course, will be very sensitive to changing customs and knowledge; and the introduction of a vaccine for measles will inevitably change its epidemic pattern, and perhaps in time eliminate the virus completely.   However, the greater understanding of epidemics that follows from appropriate models may be applied to other epidemic infections, and should assist in predicting and assessing the consequences of any changed medical practice or social customs even for measles.

PROBLEMS

1. Explain the difference between a deterministic mathematical model and a chance model.

The following problems refer to the material in small print.

2. Explain what is meant by "critical community size."

3. The deterministic model in Figure 2 predicts that there is an equilibrium point of I,S; i.e., the epidemic will never fade out. What is the concept that had to be introduced into the model to alter this prediction and thus better explain the data in Table 3 where we notice that in some communities nearly all the epidemics eventually fade-out?

4. Stated in words the formula $S_{t+1} = S_t - aI_t S_t$ says that "the number of susceptibles at the time $t+1$=number of susceptibles at time t– _____ at time t.

5. What is the equilibrium point (S_e, I_e) for the deterministic model shown in Figure 2?

6. Check by substitution that $p = 1$ and $p = Q/P$ are the solutions of the equation $p = p^2 P/(P+Q) + Q/(P+Q)$.

REFERENCES

M. S. Bartlett. 1957. "Measles Periodicity and Community Size." *Journal of the Royal Statistical Society,* A120: 48–70.

J. Graunt. 1662. Reprint, 1939. *Natural and Political Observations upon Bills of Mortality.* Baltimore: Johns Hopkins University Press.

M. Greenwood. 1935. *Epidemics and Crowd Diseases.* London: William and Norgate.

R. Ross. 1910. *The Prevention of Malaria,* Second Edition. London: J. Murray.

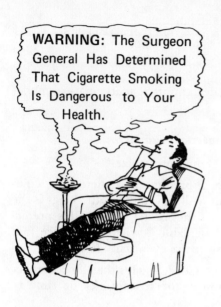

WARNING: The Surgeon General Has Determined That Cigarette Smoking Is Dangerous to Your Health.

STATISTICS, SCIENTIFIC METHOD, AND SMOKING

B. W. Brown, Jr.   *Stanford University School of Medicine*

AFTER HUNDREDS of years of tobacco use, smoking has been condemned on a scientific basis as a serious hazard to the health of the smoker. Future generations may regard the scientific indictment of smoking as a major contribution to preventive medicine and the health of the western world. Statisticians, statistical principles of scientific thought, and statistical methods of scientific study played essential parts in evaluating the effects of smoking.

Today a majority of health experts believe (though there are dissenters) that smoking is bad for the health—that it causes cancer and heart attacks and has other deleterious effects on the body. Governments have taken action to modify or suppress advertising by the tobacco industry, and to educate people about the hazards of smoking. Private health organizations, such as the American Cancer Society, actively propagandize against smoking. The effects of this new knowledge concerning smoking can readily be seen in surveys, which indicate that a growing number of people have quit smoking, that there is a decreasing proportion of smokers among young people, and that a decreasing number of cigarettes per capita are being sold. Over the last decade, the decrease in smoking at large parties, at meetings, and in public places especially among people in the health sciences, has been strikingly apparent to even casual observers.

How was it established scientifically that smoking is hazardous to the health? Why has this hazard been established only recently although smoking has been a widespread custom of the Western World for 300 years? When specific data on the question of hazard were published more than 40 years ago, why did the question spark such controversy, even among scientists most knowledgeable on the issues involved? And what role did statistics play in resolving the controversy?

EARLY VIEWS OF SMOKING AND HEALTH

Tobacco smoking is an ancient habit of man. Crude cigarettes have been found among the artifacts left by cave dwellers in Arizona; Columbus carried tobacco from the New World to the Old, with an endorsement by the Indians for its medicinal effects; Sir Walter Raleigh was a strong advocate of the use of tobacco; and many others have lauded its merits as cure and comfort for most of the diseases and distresses afflicting mankind. Cigarette smoking became so prevalent in the Western World that, according to a survey of the U.S., in the mid-sixties only 30% of males 17 years of age and older reported that they were not and had never been regular smokers. Fifty-one percent of the men and 34% of the women in the U.S. reported that they were currently regular smokers. Together, these smokers consumed more than a billion cigarettes each day in the year 1969.

Though tobacco has had its advocates from the beginning and has enjoyed an increasing, currently overwhelming popularity in the Western World, it has had opposition also, from the beginning. Swinburne said "James the First was a knave, a tyrant, a fool, a liar, a coward; but I love him, because he slit the throat of that blackguard Raleigh, who invented this filthy smoking." Some objected to the filth, while others felt the habit was sinful; still others objected that the habit was not good for the health. We can trace speculations concerning the ill effects of tobacco in records and writings as far back as three centuries, but these comments, at best, offered the authority of the experienced physician giving his impressions. They were not based on systematically gathered and evaluated scientific evidence. For example, a century ago Dr. Oliver Wendell Holmes, distinguished professor of the Harvard Medical School and father of Supreme Court Justice Holmes, said "I think tobacco often does a great deal of harm to the health. I myself gave it up many years ago." But Dr. Holmes gave no evidence to justify his conclusion.

Papers on the effects of smoking that have appeared in medical journals over the last 100 years show the general tendency of medical scientists to collect their information more systematically and to evaluate it more carefully as scientific evidence. In 1927, Dr. F. E. Tylecote, an English physician, wrote that almost every lung-cancer patient he had known about had been a regular smoker, usually of cigarettes. In 1936, Drs. Arkin and Wagner reported more specifically that 90% of 135 men afflicted with lung cancer were "chronic smokers."

DIFFICULTIES OF RESEARCH

With the accumulation of such anecdotal reports by serious medical men it became clear that the question of the harmful effects of tobacco should be subjected to scientific study. But how could the question be examined scientifically? Although scientific method in the physical sciences had been thoughtfully discussed and developed over the past several centuries, the principles that had been evolved for the physics laboratory could not be adapted easily to scientific study in the biological and medical sciences. Specifically, the biological scientist fell far short of the physicist in his attempt to hold fixed all factors except those under investigation. Instead, he was faced with investigations involving many uncontrolled, or partially controlled, factors that caused unwanted variation in the data. Conclusions had to be made in the face of this biological variation in the study material.

The problem of drawing valid scientific conclusions in the life sciences attracted an assortment of extremely able English men of science; among them were Francis Galton, a genius and creative psychologist; Karl Pearson, trained as an engineer and ultimately an outstanding philosopher of science; and R. A. Fisher, a mathematician who laid down new principles of great importance to scientific study. It was Fisher, building on the work of Galton and Pearson, who suggested, in the twenties, an alternative to the impossible requirement that all factors be held constant except the factors under investigation.

Fisher suggested that if two fertilizers, for example, are to be compared, each should be allocated to a number of different plots of ground, and that the allocation be random, according to some sort of lottery or coin-tossing system. Fisher pointed out that such random allocation would tend to balance all differences between the plots receiving the two different fertilizers and thus would yield an unbiased experiment—that is, one fair to both fertilizers. He further pointed out that any differences in the results obtained with the two fertilizers could be evaluated, using the probability theory that had been developed for gambling games, to decide how likely it was that so large a difference might have come about simply through a chance allocation of the more fertile plots to one of the treatments.

This new scientific methodology, employing randomization and probability theory, was a tremendous contribution to the young science of statistics. It spread quickly through the agricultural sciences and then ·to the medical sciences. Today a new drug will not be approved by the U.S. Food and Drug Administration for marketing until it has been compared with other treatments in what is called a *randomized clinical trial*. In the thirties, however, these rigorous standards for scientific study were new and scientists were just becoming familiar with their application in the medical sciences. How could the new methodology be applied to the smoking question?

RETROSPECTIVE STUDIES

Clearly it would be difficult, though perhaps not impossible, to conduct a randomized experiment on human beings to determine whether smoking is harmful. The first attempt at some sort of satisfactory substitute approach was to identify cases of lung cancer and, at the same time, to select some other persons comparable to the lung-cancer patients in age, sex, and other characteristics, and then to determine whether the persons with lung cancer smoked more heavily than the artificially constructed "control group." The first study of this kind was reported by Müller in 1939, who found much more smoking among the lung-cancer cases. Of course, it was clear to statisticians and others that this kind of data must be regarded with caution. The "control group" in such a study can only be selected somewhat arbitrarily and it is quite easy to imagine that the selection might tend to omit, or fail to recognize, smokers because of conscious or unconscious bias on the part of either the investigator or the persons responding to questions regarding their own smoking habits or those of their deceased relatives. Similarly, biases might exaggerate smoking experience among the lung-cancer cases.

Because the retrospective approach did not measure up to the standards of the randomized clinical experiment, other approaches were tried. Raymond Pearl (1938), an eminent medical statistician at Johns Hopkins University, had been keeping close records of health experiences of hundreds of families in the Baltimore area for some years. Pearl's work was going on at the time that serious study of the tobacco and health question began, and he decided to compile information about the smoking habits and longevity of all males in his files. Using the statistical methods common in computing life tables for life insurance purposes, Professor Pearl constructed a life table for nonsmokers, another for moderate smokers and a third for heavy smokers (see Figure 1). His data showed that 65% of the nonsmokers survive to age 60, whereas only 45% of the heavy smokers live that long. Indeed, Figure 1 shows that at every age between 30 and 90, proportionately more nonsmokers survive

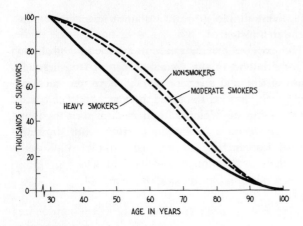

FIGURE 1

*The survivorship lines of life
tables for white males falling
into three categories relative to
their tobacco usage: (a) nonsmokers, (b) moderate smokers,
smokers, and (c) heavy smokers.
Source: Pearl (1938)*

than moderate smokers, who, in turn, survive longer than heavy smokers.
The impressive study hinted at smoking effects far beyond an increase in
the relatively rare disease of lung cancer.

When Pearl's results were published, they added substantial weight to
the evidence against smoking. But his claims were based on a special kind
of study, so workers who did not have this sort of longitudinal data continued
using the retrospective method of identifying lung-cancer patients and demon-
strating that these patients were tobacco smokers to a much larger extent
than any comparable control group that might be chosen. In the next decade
many such retrospective studies were published, but the mounting number
of scientific reports did not add conviction in proportion to their number.
They all used the same method and they all might be drawing the same
erroneous conclusion. Meanwhile, the consumption of tobacco per capita
continued to increase, smoking among teenagers continued to rise, and the
medical profession as a whole did not advise the public against the habit.

Medical scientists recognized the tremendous importance of the question.
Tobacco was an intimate and welcome part of the lives of a substantial portion
of the people. The tobacco industry was a vital part of the economy of
a huge region of the U. S. and furnished the livelihood of additional thousands
through related industries such as advertising, transportation, and sales. If
tobacco were as harmful as Pearl's 1938 paper indicated, it would be the

obligation of the medical profession and government health agencies to help the public protect itself against this hazard.   On the other hand, if the studies were erroneous, it would be extremely unfortunate if the medical profession or the government were to interfere in private lives and disrupt large segments of the economy on the basis of unsound scientific work.   Thus medical scientists were deeply concerned about assessing the strength of the evidence against tobacco.   Statisticians, especially in the biological and medical sciences, found themselves at the center of the dilemma facing the question.   "Is the retrospective study a sound scientific approach?"

PROSPECTIVE STUDIES

It was felt that a new kind of study—more closely resembling the randomized clinical study—must be done.   Pearl's choice of subjects and study were unsatisfactory in that his methods for choosing families and for choosing subjects within the families were never clearly set down.   The chance for substantial biases in selection of the subjects and in the interviews for smoking experience seemed unacceptably large, and the report was not taken seriously.   His prospective approach, however, in which smokers and nonsmokers are identified and then studied until death is an appealing one.   It is a much closer approximation of a real experiment, in which a population would be split randomly into two groups; one group would be given one treatment (in this case, smoking) and the other group would receive an alternative treatment (no smoking).   Both groups would be studied over time to determine the effects of the treatments.   Even in the prospective study, the lack of random assignment of persons to be smokers and nonsmokers means that the conclusions are subject to the reservation that the smokers may be different from the nonsmokers in some systematic way that is entirely unrelated to their smoking habits, but that is causally related to some other factor that is deleterious to their health. For example, suppose that people who *like* smoking tend to get cancer and people who *don't like* it tend not to. Despite this inherent weakness in the prospective study approach, statisticians and other scientists called for this kind of study, and several were conducted in the fifties.

The first two prospective studies of the tobacco question were done by eminent statisticians in England and the U.S. In England, Dr. Richard Doll and Sir A. Bradford Hill, whose careful retrospective studies of the question had led them to conclude that smoking does cause lung cancer, were the first to report on a prospective study. They sent questionnaires to all members of the medical profession in the United Kingdom, roughly 60,000 men and women, and received about 40,000 replies. They asked about present smoking habits and a few other characteristics, such as age and sex. Then, through the Registrars-General in the United Kingdom, they determined the survivorship of these men and women over a period of several years. Their study results were as anticipated: there were remarkably more lung-cancer deaths among the smokers than among the nonsmokers. Of course, this report, based on a different study approach in which the information on smoking habits was obtained first, rather than after the fact of death or disease, was regarded as extremely important additional evidence against smoking.

The prospective study offered new information that could not be obtained from the retrospective study. The retrospective study offered counts of smokers among lung-cancer cases. The prospective study offered counts of lung-cancer deaths among smokers and, thus, a direct measure of the death rate for lung cancer among smokers. The Doll and Hill data showed the rate for heavy smokers to be 1.66 per 1000 men per year, compared to 0.07 for nonsmokers; thus, heavy smokers had a lung-cancer death rate 24 times higher than nonsmokers. But even more important, the prospective study recorded all deaths and the recorded causes of these deaths, whereas the retrospective studies focused on the cause of death that was suspect. With information on all deaths that occurred in the group it was found that there was also a surplus of deaths due to heart attack among the smokers, and that this surplus was not readily explainable as chance variation in the data. Medical investigators had reported the effects of tobacco on the body (for example, the immediate cooling of the skin through contraction of the blood vessels when a person begins to smoke a cigarette), but the Doll and Hill study provided rather direct evidence that such effects on the heart and blood system could increase the risk of early death. The death rate for heart attacks among smokers was 5.99 per 1000 men per year for heavy smokers and 4.22 for nonsmokers—not a large difference, but extremely important, if real, because of the large number of deaths from this cause.

The second prospective study was reported by two American statisticians, Dr. E. Cuyler Hammond and Dr. Daniel Horn. Through the American Cancer Society, these men enlisted the aid of about 22,000 woman volunteers, each of whom was asked to select 10 healthy men between the ages of 50 and 69 and have each of them fill out a smoking questionnaire. Then these women reported on the health status of each of these men each year. Death certificates were obtained for each death reported. About 200,000 men were followed through a period of almost four years during which some 12,000 of them died. The Hammond and Horn report confirmed the findings of the Doll and Hill prospective study. Hammond and Horn reported a lung-cancer rate 23.4 times higher among heavy smokers (more than one pack a day) compared to nonsmokers and a death rate for heart and circulatory diseases 1.57 times as high among heavy smokers as among nonsmokers. Hammond and Horn emphasized the fact that although lung-cancer rates were strikingly high among smokers, the greater share of the excess deaths among smokers occurred in the heart and circulatory disease category, simply because this is a much more common cause of death.

NEW OBJECTIONS

Further prospective studies, involving different investigators and large groups of subjects chosen from various sources and followed for periods of up to a decade, were reported in the late fifties and early sixties. All of these studies substantiated the results of the first two studies. The evidence, which had been carefully gathered and evaluated by eminent men of medicine and statistics, seemed to condemn tobacco. But two factors were yet to be reckoned with: the impressive economic importance of tobacco as a prime industry and as contributor to other industries and the overwhelming strength of the smoking habit among the population. Again the statisticians played a major role in the drama, but this time, surprisingly, their influence was in defense of the "vile weed." One of the defenders was Sir Ronald Fisher, the man whose ideas were behind the randomized clinical trial and perhaps the greatest statistician who ever lived (Fisher died in the mid-sixties). Another statistician who came to the defense of tobacco was Dr. Joseph Berkson, Chief of Medical Statistics for the famed Mayo Clinic until he retired in the mid-sixties and one of the most creative people in medical statistics, having been trained in both medicine and medical statistics. Fisher and Berkson, both colorful and persuasive scientists, in the past had often found themselves on opposite sides of arguments concerning scientific methodology. This time they were on the same side, however, and Berkson was heard to say in jest that this was the only point that caused him serious doubt about his position on the tobacco-health question.

Although the positions taken by Fisher and Berkson gave aid and comfort to the habitual smoker, to the tobacco industry, and to the people who made their living through the tobacco industry, it must be stressed that these men had a larger and more important issue in mind, namely, the methodology of science itself. And, though the short-term effect of their writings was a delay in the scientific indictment of tobacco, the long-term effects will more than counterbalance these by tightening up scientific standards for medical studies in which appropriate randomized clinical experiments cannot be carried out because of possible danger to participants. In the late fifties, Fisher and Berkson both repeatedly pointed out that the evidence against tobacco as a hazard to the health was only circumstantial because clinical experiments could not be done. They pointed out, in detail, weaknesses in the evidence, even in the evidence from the prospective studies. They proposed other explanations that would account for the data if tobacco had no deleterious effects on the health.

Berkson's main point was that the apparent ill effects of smoking were too pervasive. The death rates seemed to be higher for too many different causes of death. Such a universally bad effect from tobacco was never anticipated, and there were no theories to explain how smoking could cause death through each of the multitude of diseases implicated by the reports from the prospective studies. Berkson suggested that a more likely explanation was that there were biases in sample selection, or in the data collected, or both, and that these biases affected all of the prospective studies because they were inherent in the methodology of the prospective studies and they affected all causes of death. Otherwise, Berkson suggested, we must hypothesize some sort of general constitutional effect of smoking on the body, or some sort of accelerated aging caused by smoking; he was dissatisfied also by the absence of known mechanisms causing the disorders.

Fisher, who had been knighted for his work in genetics and who had always been concerned with the problems of interpreting nonexperimental (i.e., nonrandomized) studies, put these two interests together and argued that if persons with a hereditary tendency toward smoking also had a hereditary predilection for disease, the result would be exactly the kind that had been repeatedly demonstrated, both retrospectively and prospectively. Then, Fisher argued, if the explanation lay in such hereditary predilections, a smoker who quit could not change his genetic makeup or his peculiar higher risk of disease thereby, and smoking could not be regarded as harmful to health. Fisher proposed some (nonrandomized) twin studies that might shed light on his hypotheses, but little could be done because large groups of people were needed for definitive results. (See the essay by Reid, especially Table 2 and its discussion.)

Neither Fisher nor Berkson has been completely answered. In fact, the questions they raised cannot be answered definitively without randomized experiments. Of course, Fisher and Berkson knew this as well as anyone, but such conspicuous critiques, made by widely known men of high prestige, in the context of a scientific question of intense public interest, served to underline the dangers in drawing conclusions from nonrandomized studies.

FURTHER RESEARCH

The immediate effect of the Fisher and Berkson critiques was to spur on statisticians and medical scientists to an even more careful look at the tobacco-health question. Although the questions raised by Berkson and Fisher could never be answered directly, additional indirect evidence has been marshaled on many points. There is space here only to mention some of the approaches, without detailing their results.

Because experimental verification of smoking as a cause of ill effects in man did not seem practicable, scientists had attempted to investigate the effects of tobacco smoke on animals, where random assignment to smoking and nonsmoking groups was feasible. Although much experimental work had been done, until the early sixties the actual smoking experience of the human had not been adequately simulated in the laboratory and no direct positive evidence had been obtained. In the sixties, however, studies demonstrated that tobacco smoke and some of its constituents do cause lesions in animal tissue that are similar to those seen in human lung cancer. When, finally, an experimental setup was attained that satisfactorily simulated the smoking habit in dogs, a few cases of lung cancer were induced in what seemed to be well-controlled, randomized experiments.

At the same time, in partial answer to Berkson's point that there was no theory or information that would lead one to suspect that smoking would affect the diversity of organs and systems cited in the prospective reports, much work in animals and humans has been carried out to determine what physiological effects tobacco has on the organ systems. One of the most important results has been the discovery that tobacco smoke does have deleterious effects on the blood vessels of animals and the verification of this same damage in the blood vessels of heavy smokers.

The evidence against tobacco has been strengthened by more detailed information and closer statistical evaluation in ongoing prospective studies. It has been found that smoking is not associated with all causes of death, but that for the causes implicated, the death rates increase regularly and convincingly with the amount smoked. When the details of smoking habits and smoking experience were analyzed, including especially the results for persons who had smoked but quit the habit for varying lengths of time, the death rates have been found to be closely consistent with what might be expected if smoking were indeed a causal factor in death.

THE SURGEON GENERAL'S REPORT

By the mid-sixties, scientific opinion had swung far toward the conclusion that smoking is harmful. Despite the realization that the evidence against smoking can only be indirect, scientists were convinced that some conclusion must be reached and acted on for the good of the public health. A special committee, appointed by the Surgeon General of the U.S. Public Health Service, made a long and thorough study of all aspects of the tobacco-health question. The committee of ten men included experts on chemistry, pharmacology, internal medicine, surgery, pathology, epidemiology, and statistics. The statistical representative was William G. Cochran, Professor of Statistics at Harvard University and a world-renowned expert in the application of statistical methodology to problems of the life sciences. In 1963 this Advisory Committee submitted to the Surgeon General a report that cited smoking as a cause of lung cancer and several other cancers and stated that the evidence pointing to smoking as a cause of death due to heart attack was strong enough to justify acting on this presumption.

LATER DEVELOPMENTS

In the sixties, independent health organizations and governmental health agencies in this country and throughout the world publicly announced their conclusions that tobacco is a health hazard. Along with these indictments came a call for further action. Many health officials felt that it wasn't enough to inform the public through the usual scientific publications, carried along by brief news reports and by word of mouth. Rather, they felt that a public habituated to tobacco and under constant bombardment by advertisements that associated cigarettes with youth, health, attractiveness, and elegance must be protected. The issue became one of how far the responsibility and legal authority of the government can extend to protect the citizen against himself and against the influences of deleterious propaganda, especially when the evidence did not measure up to the standards of true experimental science.

By 1970, there were still scientists (a few of them statisticians) who found the evidence against smoking less than convincing and who were willing to so testify at congressional hearings. But, for the most part, statisticians will play a new part in the tobacco-health arena as the issue ceases to be a question of science and becomes one of public policy. In 1969, Bernard Greenberg, Professor of Biostatistics at the University of North Carolina and a noted public health statistician, published a paper discussing the strength of evidence against smoking and the extent to which such evidence might justify various levels of government action in protection of the individual. These possible actions ranged from rather modest propaganda campaigns to legal judgments against tobacco companies for causing untimely death and illness through the vending of their product. Professor Greenberg's paper was not a philosophical discussion, concerned with ethical, political, and legal principles; it was an attempt to use modern statistical theory—this time a branch of mathematical statistics called *decision theory*—to arrive at reasoned advice, based on the costs to the public of actions that might be taken and the gains and losses that might accrue to the public as the result of such actions. This new kind of thinking in public health requires a different kind of statistical theory than that for experiments.

SUMMARY

This essay has traced the role of some eminent statisticians and the statistical methods they used to determine that smoking is harmful to the public health. The work that has been done on this problem and the debates on scientific method that it has stimulated will have untold benefit both through the eventual elimination of smoking as a general habit of the people and in the development of better techniques and higher standards for the scientific study of other hazards to the public health in the future.

PROBLEMS

1. What did R. A. Fisher suggest to use as an alternative to holding all factors constant except the ones under investigation?

2. Explain what is meant by an "unbiased experiment."

3. Explain the terms "retrospective study" and "prospective study." Give the pros and cons.

4. Refer to Figure 1. Approximately what percentage of males survived up to age 50 in the three different categories?

5. Refer to Figure 1. What was the approximate median lifetime (i.e., the age up to which 50% of the people survived) in each of the three categories?

6. What were the objections of Berkson and Fisher to the results of both the prospective and retrospective studies?

7. If a prospective study shows that there is a higher incidence of lung cancer among smokers than among nonsmokers, can we conclude that smoking causes lung cancer? Why or why not?

REFERENCES

Joseph Berkson. 1958. "Smoking and Lung Cancer: Some Observations on Two Recent Reports." *Journal of the American Statistical Association* 53:28–38.

Harold Diehl. 1970. *Tobacco and Your Health: The Smoking Controversy.* New York: McGraw-Hill.

Alfred Dunhill. 1954. *The Gentle Art of Smoking.* New York: Putnam.

R. A. Fisher. 1959. *Smoking: The Cancer Controversy.* Edinburgh: Oliver & Boyd.

B. G. Greenberg. 1969. "Problems of Statistical Inference in Health with Special Reference to the Cigarette Smoking and Lung Cancer Controversy." *Journal of the American Statistical Association* 64:739–758.

A. E. Hamilton. 1927. *This Smoking World.* New York: Appleton–Century.

Raymond Pearl. 1938. "Tobacco Smoking and Longevity." *Science* 87:216–217.

U. S. Public Health Service. 1963. *Smoking and Health.* Report of the Advisory Committee to the Surgeon General.

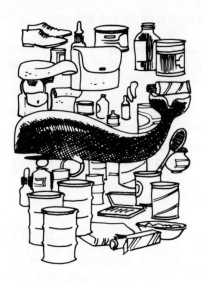

THE PLIGHT OF THE WHALES

D. G. Chapman   *University of Washington*

BETWEEN THE end of World War I and 1960, several species of whales in the ocean around the Antarctic continent were the basis of an important industry. These giant mammals, the largest that have ever existed on the earth, were sought for animal oil and, to a lesser extent, meal and meat extract (the latter for human consumption) as well as a myriad of byproducts. In antiquity, whalers went out in small boats and endured great risks to capture such large sources of meat. Men continued to hunt whales in small boats with primitive weapons, as portrayed in *Moby Dick,* until late in the nineteenth century. In the twentieth century, whaling has been highly modernized with explosive harpoons, large ships, and powerful radar-equipped catcher boats, which enable the whaling industry to operate in the stormy and inhospitable oceans next to the Antarctic ice cap.

This area of the world, while unfriendly to man, is very inviting to whales, for during the southern summer the waters bloom with small plants which, in turn, feed myriads of minute animals, known generally as *krill*. Certain species of whales catch these by straining large volumes of water in their huge mouths through sievelike filters called *baleen plates* (hence this group of whales is referred to as baleen whales). These whales have no teeth and do not eat fish or other marine mammals. The largest of the baleen whales, and indeed of all whales, are the blue whales, which may reach a length of 100 feet, though 70 to 80 feet is a more usual size.

BLUE WHALES

Immediately following World War II, Europe and Japan were in desperate need of many things, including animal oil. It was not surprising, therefore, that the number of Antarctic whaling catcher boats increased; furthermore, technologies developed during the War made whaling more efficient. As a result, some conservationists feared that Antarctic whales, particularly the blue whales, would be completely eliminated. Figure 1 shows the annual catch of blue whales in the southern oceans in the decade before the War and in the postwar period to 1960. The basis for concern for the blue whales was easy to document, but the catch of other species was stable or increasing. Some of those associated with the industry suggested reasons other than a decline in population for the decline of the blue whale catch and were re-

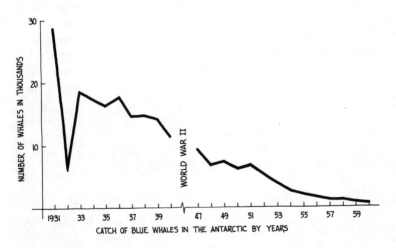

FIGURE 1

Catch of blue whales in the Antarctic, seasons 1930–31 to 1959–60 excluding World War II period

luctant to accept restrictions on catches. Thus the International Whaling Commission, set up in 1946 to manage the resource, found itself the center of controversy. The Commission has representatives from all interested countries; it establishes size regulations and quotas, and also has the authority to ban hunting of species that appear to be endangered.

The Commission set up a study group to bring together all the data and develop statistical methods for attacking such questions as: How many whales are in the stock that feed in the Antarctic? How many young are born each year? How many whales die from natural causes each year? How are these birth and death rates affected by factors over which man has some control?

COUNTING METHODS

Let us consider the first, and perhaps most basic, question: How many whales are there of a particular species? Whales unfortunately don't stay still to be counted. They roam over large areas, spending most of their time under water, though they do surface at regular intervals to breathe. Furthermore, the southern oceans cover a vast part of the world; the whaling area exceeds 10 million square miles, an area larger than all of North America.

Marking Method. There are several standard ways to estimate wild animal populations, all of which involve some statistical techniques. We shall describe three of them. The first involves marking a number of whales; a foot-long metal cylinder is fired into the thick blubber that lies just under the skin. If and when marked whales are later caught, some information is available on their movement, on their rate of capture, and on the proportion of marked members in the whole herd. The usefulness of the latter information is easily seen by simulating such an experiment with a can of marbles. Assume that like the whale population, the number of marbles in the can is unknown. Now pick a few marbles (say, ten) out of the can, mark them, and return them to the can. Next, stir the whole can thoroughly and draw another sample. Count separately the marked and unmarked marbles. If the unmarked ones are four times as numerous in the sample as the marked ones, we reason that the same is true of the whole canful; but because there is a total of ten marked marbles, we infer there are 40 unmarked marbles, or 50 marbles in total.

This simple scheme has been used with many animal populations, though there are many obvious complications in practice, and for whales this is especially true. How do we know, for example, that the metal mark fired into the blubber actually penetrated and did not ricochet off? Did the crew who cut up the captured whale carefully look for the mark—even a foot-long metal cylinder is easy to overlook in cold, stormy working conditions when the volume being cut up is approximately the size of a house. Also, unlike the marbles, whales are born and die over a period of years. All of these complications require refinements and extensions of the simple experiment outlined here. It is necessary to have a series of experiments extending over many years and to use comparative procedures. For example, if a group of whales is marked in year 1 and a group of the same size is marked in year 2, then, after year 2, the ratio of recoveries of whales marked in year 1 to the recoveries of whales marked in year 2 reflects the proportion of marked whales of group 1 that died in the intervening year. These deaths may have been natural or caused by hunters. Moreover, the *ratio* is a valid measure of this mortality because its numerator and denominator are equally affected by the possible errors listed above. Such a comparative study is only one of the several statistical procedures used to analyze whale-marking data.

Catch-per-Day Method. The second estimation method is based on changes in the rate of catching whales. The rate of catching depends mainly on the frequency with which whales are seen, and other things being equal, this depends on their density. Thus the catch per day reflects the density. How can this be translated into absolute numbers? If the change in catch per day is entirely a result of the removal by man, then it is easy to make this translation; if catching 25,000 whales in one season lowers the catch rate for the next season by 10% then at the outset of the first season there must have been 25,000/0.10, or 250,000 whales.

Again, the situation is more complex than this simple example. Whaling ships hunt over a vast area in difficult conditions, so that the catches fluctuate violently. Whaling companies introduce new technology to improve their efficiency. Moreover, we reemphasize that there are other causes of whale mortality, and that there are new births as well; both of these factors must be taken into account in adjusting the population estimate. One way to overcome some of these difficulties is to adjust for changes in efficiency and also to follow the change in catch per day (adjusted) over a period of several seasons. Figure 2 shows the catch per day of blue whales plotted against the cumulative catch by the whaling-factory ships over the seasons 1953–54 to 1962–63 when natural deaths and births were numerically quite small. As more whales were caught, the catch per day went steadily down. This graph suggests that there were only 10,000–12,000 blue whales in 1953 and this number declined to about 1000 in 1963. As pointed out, there are statistical refinements, and the result obtained in this way must be combined with estimates obtained in other ways.

Age Analysis. The catch-per-day method works well with rapidly declining populations, but in other situations, the complications and corrections make it less useful. Still a third method is available, however, that uses the ages of whales. Just as trees have annual rings in their trunks and fish have

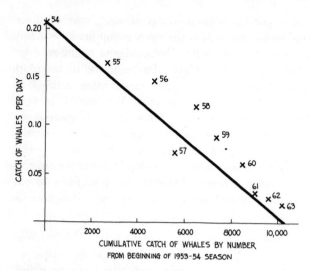

FIGURE 2

Blue whale catch per day (adjusted for efficiency improvements) versus cumulative catch, 1953–54 to 1962–63

annual rings in their scales, whales have annual rings in a waxy secretion in the ear (earplugs). The ages of a sample of the whales killed each year were determined by the rings of their earplugs. In addition, information on the length of every whale killed commercially made it possible to relate age to length and to calculate an estimated age for every captured whale.

It was thus possible to make a statistical estimation of the number of four-year-old whales in any season and the number of five-year-olds in the following season. Because one year's five-year-olds are the survivors of the previous year's four-year-olds, a survival rate or, conversely, a mortality rate can be determined. Because all ages are estimated and because some adjustments have to be made, the estimated mortality rates fluctuate wildly. However, by averaging over several year's classes, over areas and seasons, useful results can be obtained. Furthermore, with additional statistical analysis, it is even possible to assess the magnitudes of possible errors in such estimations. These mortality rates help us to predict the future of the whale population. (See the essay by Keyfitz for an explanation of this method as applied to human populations.)

Results. Thus we have three methods of estimating population sizes and mortality rates: the marking method, the catch-per-day method, and age analysis. The results of different methods were checked against one another, and fortunately the different estimates were in good agreement. Sources of error were carefully checked and ruled out, so that the study group finally concluded that the blue whales numbered at most a few thousand and might total even less than 1000. Thus there was and is a real danger of extinction of this species in the Antarctic (there are also small numbers of blue whales in the northern oceans). Fortunately, the International Whaling Commission banned the taking of blue whales as soon as the study was finished—first, in a large párt of the southern oceans and eventually in all waters south of the equator. It is too soon to predict the long-term survival of the species; blue whales are occasionally seen, but these are probably the survivors noted above (whales can live, in the absence of hunting, to more than 40 years of age). We can ask whether the population has been reduced to such low levels that reproduction is reduced below the level necessary for species continuation, but it will be a number of years before this can be answered.

FIN WHALES

The second-largest whale species in the world, also part of the baleen family, is the fin whale. It averages about ten feet less than the blue whale in length. During the fifties this stock annually yielded in excess of one million barrels of oil per year. With the decline of the blue whales, fin whales bore the brunt of the exploitation. The same methods of analysis used for the blue whales were applied to the fin whales; in fact, the analysis was more critically needed because the condition of the fin whale stock was not obvious as was that of the blue whales. Moreover, fin whale catches were still very high: in the 1961–62 season over 27,000 fin whales were killed. The study group recommended that the fin whale catch should be reduced to 7000, or less, if the fin whale stock was not to be further depleted. The proposal for such a drastic reduction came as a shock to the Commission; the study group forecast that the next season's catch, regardless of quotas, would drop to 14,000. When actual figures proved the forecast right, most countries wanted to move toward the drastic reductions required, but some of the whaling nations were able to block action. Another disastrous season caused a revision in the thinking of the commissioners, and in 1965, a substantial schedule of reductions in the quota was agreed upon. Nevertheless, the delay in reaching this agreement and the delay in reducing the quota subsequently, meant that the presently permitted catches have had to be lowered even further. Subsequent analyses using additional data show that, as of 1971, catches in excess of 3000 per year are likely to mean further reduction of the stock. This drastic reduction in the permitted catch has had a severe impact on the industry. Of the five countries that hunted whales with factory ships in the Antarctic in 1960, only Japan and the Soviet Union are still actively engaged in the industry. Further, these have diverted some of their effort to catching smaller whales of little interest in other times and have transferred some factory ships to other oceans or to other types of fishing.

THE FUTURE OF THE WHALE STOCK

The study group was asked to advise the Commission not only on the state of the whale stocks, but also on what the optimum stock size might be. The optimum size is that which will yield the maximum number of whales each year on a continuing basis. It is now recognized that whales should be managed like our fisheries and forestry resources on a sustained-yield basis. So far, no one has found a way of harvesting the plankton production of the southern oceans except via the whales. In 1969, the Soviet Union sent a ship to the Antarctic waters to harvest the krill directly. They succeeded in catching a reasonable quantity, which they converted to a krill paste, reported to be quite tasty. Unfortunately, to meet the costs involved, they were forced to sell it on the Moscow market at about the same price as beef. Faced with a choice between beef and krill paste, the Moscow housewife did exactly what her Western counterpart would do, so the krill harvest was a failure.

The whale stocks should be allowed to increase because the statistical analysis shows that the optimum levels are much higher than the present depleted stock sizes. The steps to permit stocks to increase are difficult, but at least the Commission has now fully accepted the methods of analysis that were first applied to whales in this study. The present quota on catches, not only in southern oceans but also in the North Pacific, is based on the best scientific evidence as reviewed and analyzed by the Scientific Committee of the Whaling Commission, which includes scientists (particularly experts in population statistics) from Canada, Great Britain, Japan, Norway, the Soviet Union, and the U.S., as well as the Food and Agriculture Organization of the United Nations. One loophole remains: each whaling country has the responsibility for enforcing the quota and other restrictions without any supervision by international observers. Steps are being taken to change this. It is to be deplored that scientific methods were not introduced sooner and that even now stricter enforcement is necessary, but recent restrictions by the Commission represent a major accomplishment in management of a world resource, one that will survive only if man and nations cooperate to save it.

PROBLEMS

1. Refer to Figure 1. What was the approximate catch of blue whales in the Antarctic in the season 1931–32? 1937–38? What is the percentage reduction between the two seasons? When was the catch the highest? The lowest?

2. What are the three counting methods discussed in the text? Describe briefly.

3. Describe an experiment whose purpose is to estimate the size of a human population in an isolated island, using one of the methods mentioned in the article. What assumptions are you making?

4. Refer to Figure 2. What was the approximate catch of blue whales per day (adjusted) in the season 1955–56 (plotted as 1956)?

5. Refer to Figure 2. Can you explain the relative "high" for the 1958 figure?

6. From Figure 2 it was concluded that there were only 10,000–12,000 blue whales in 1953. How was this number obtained?

7. Suppose it was determined by the age analysis method that the mortality rate of blue whales is .25 per year. Furthermore by the marking method it was estimated that there were about 7000 blue whales at the start of 1960. How many whales would you expect to be still living at the end of 1961 assuming that the mortality rate does not change over the years?

8. What is meant by "optimum stock size" of whales? Why should there be an optimum size at all?

REFERENCES

D. G. Chapman, K. R. Allen, and S. J. Holt. 1964. "Reports of the Committee of Three Scientists on the Special Antarctic Investigations of the Antarctic Whale Stocks." *Fourteenth Report of the International Whaling Commission.* London. Pp. 32–106.

J. A. Gulland. 1966. "The Effect of Regulation on Antarctic Whale Catches." *Journal du Conseil,* 30:308–315.

N. A. Mackintosh. 1965. *The Stocks of Whales.* London: Fishing News.

Scott McVay. 1966. "The Last of the Great Whales." *Scientific American,* 215:2, pp. 13–21.

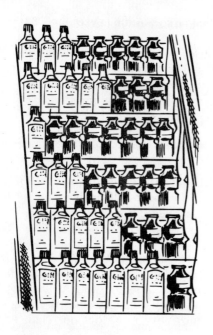

SETTING DOSAGE LEVELS

W. J. Dixon   *University of California, Los Angeles*

MANY OF the problems brought to the statistician for solution require pinpointing a level at which an expected response does or does not occur in order to test the strength and efficacy of drugs, pesticides, hormones, explosives, analgesics, stimulants, fuels, and a wide variety of other materials important to man and his environment. A statistician feels particularly successful if he develops a method for solving such problems that has a wide range of applications. One such method is called the *up-and-down,* or *staircase, method.* This is the way it works.

HOW STRONG SHOULD PUNCH BE?

Mr. and Mrs. Smith, aged 22 and 20, respectively, are planning their first cocktail party, inviting all of the people in Mr. Smith's office. They can't afford an elaborate party, but they do want to make a good impression, so they have decided to serve a punch made of gin and cranberry juice. They have little experience with alcohol, and so they don't know the proportion of gin to cranberry juice; they decide to try the punch first on some reliable and courageous friends. Four couples agree to help out.

Mr. Smith thinks all the guests will want at least 8 ounces of punch. Mrs. Smith wants her guests to be happy, but doesn't want anyone to become ill at her party. This is where the courageous friends (guinea pigs) come in. Mr. Smith mixes the first drink with 7 ounces of gin and 1 ounce of cranberry juice, and Mr. Big tosses it down. In about half an hour he is green and staggering. Obviously the punch contained too little cranberry juice. The next drink, 5 ounces of gin to 3 ounces of cranberry juice, goes to Mr. Jones. He is still on his feet half an hour later, but he is behaving strangely. Mrs. Big decides she will be safer if she volunteers for the 3-to-5 mixture. This turns out to be a mistake because she soon feels very warm. Mr. Smith refuses to let Mrs. Smith have a drink, and he believes that he himself must stay out of the testing to keep the record straight. The 1-to-7 drink, therefore, goes to Mr. Average who compliments his hostess on the delicious flavor, but says he really doesn't feel a thing. Mr. Small thinks he should have something stronger and asks for 5 ounces of gin to 3 ounces of cranberry juice. Mr. Small suddenly develops a slight speech defect, so the next drink is again made 3 to 5, and Mrs. Average drinks it. She compliments the hostess, saying the drink is excellent. She is happy and relaxed. Mrs. Small asks for a drink with the same proportions, and the Smiths thank their friends for having solved the problem. They will serve punch made from 3 parts gin and 5 parts cranberry juice.

The basic notion illustrated in this simple example is that of moving some important control level up or down each time, depending on the prior level and the outcome of the prior trial. In the example, when the response of the experimenters suggested too much alcohol, the dose was reduced for the next trial. When the response suggested too little alcohol, the dose was increased. In the end, some judgment was made as to final level. What sort of problems can be easily solved by this method?

APPRAISING STRENGTHS OF OTHER MATERIALS

Some drugs are grown naturally, and they must be tested to determine how strong they are. Penicillin is an example. Most hormones must be similarly assayed for their strength.

(1) Pesticides should be strong enough to destroy insects, but not poison the family cat.

(2) Pain killers should relieve headaches, but not induce palpitations.

(3) Jet propulsion engines must have explosive-type "motors" capable of propelling an airplane, but the explosions must not shake the vehicle to pieces.

How can we design a measurement process that gives us sufficient assurance that we are arriving at a correct dose of a drug, one that will do what is desired? How can we do this in an efficient manner?

In order to test the strength of any given material, we must set up some standard of potency, or performance. With poisons, it is customary to use test animals of similar size and heredity and to inject each with a known concentration of the drug to be studied. A widely used, though arbitrary, choice is that the standard, or threshold, will be that concentration which will kill, on the average, half the animals tested. Obviously, other levels may be used, but if we understand how to handle one level, we are well along toward handling others. Let us examine in detail such a problem and one method for dealing with it.

Curare, a poison that paralyzes the heart and motor-nerve endings in striated muscle, was used for thousands of years by primitive people to destroy their enemies. Doctors now use this lethal substance for the benefit of mankind in certain surgical and medical procedures. Another poison with similar properties is the venom of the scorpion fish. To use this venom properly, we must have a precise measure of the strength of any batch we plan to use. Scorpion fish venom, in fact, has been assayed by the up-and-down method. This is how we went about setting up the trials.

APPRAISING SCORPION FISH VENOM USING FIXED SAMPLE SIZES

An amount of the venom (the stimulus) will be injected into test animals (in this case, mice), and we will record whether a response (death) occurs in a given time period, say, 30 minutes. If we have chosen a dose that is too large, all (or almost all) the animals will die. If the dose is too small, possibly none of the animals will die. How can we find the dose that corresponds to the amount of poison that, if increased, causes more than half of the animals, on the average, to die and, if decreased, causes fewer than half to die? Even if he lives, the same animal cannot be used in a second test because he now may be less able or more able to stand the venom. The task would still not be very difficult if all animals behaved in the same way. Even in carefully selected animals, however, the amount of a drug required to bring about a response differs greatly from animal to animal. The amount of a drug just sufficient to cause a response in a particular animal is called his *threshold level*. We want to estimate some sort of average threshold for the population of animals.

Our measurement for a particular animal given a certain dose will be a response (in this case, death), which we shall record as "X," or a non-response, which will be recorded as "O."

How do we decide on the dose (stimulus) to give each animal? If an individual's threshold is unaffected by the test, we could merely increase a single animal's stimulus gradually until the threshold is reached. Unfortunately, this is not the case; estimating a mean threshold requires careful experimental design.

How can we attack this problem in an efficient manner? One natural design gives an experiment in which the same number of animals are tested at each of a variety of dose levels. To introduce some order into this situation we choose four different dose levels (say, 1, 2, 4, 8 mg) of venom. (It turns out that dosages of a wide variety of chemicals show approximately uniform increments in effectiveness if each dose is a certain percent larger than the preceding dose, i.e., if doses are chosen so that each is a multiple of the preceding one. In our example the doses increase by factors of 2.) We test five mice at each level. If we are so unlucky as to have picked a set of dosages that are all clearly below the threshold of all animals, we learn nothing about the location of the threshold for these animals except that it is greater than the largest dose given, 8 mg. We don't know how much greater. Or, if all animals at all levels respond, we discover only that the threshold is below the smallest dose, 1 mg. Even if the set of dosage levels chosen covers the general threshold level, we may test at a number of doses to which all or none of the animals respond.

Table 1 and Figure 1 show a set of outcomes from such a procedure. Five animals were tested at each of four dosage levels, with the outcomes as shown. Twenty animals were required.

SEQUENTIAL TESTING: THE UP-AND-DOWN METHOD

It is only common sense to seek a testing strategy that leads the experimenter quickly to the proper levels for the tests. We wish to destroy as few mice

TABLE 1. Outcomes for Five Animals at Each Dosage Level in the Order in Which They Are Treated (X Means Death; O Means Survival)

DOSAGE LEVELS	OUTCOMES				
8 mg	X	X	X	X	X
4 mg	X	X	O	X	X
2 mg	O	O	X	X	O
1 mg	O	O	O	O	O

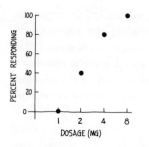

FIGURE 1

Data of Table 1 plotted to show relation between response rate (percent dying) and dosage level

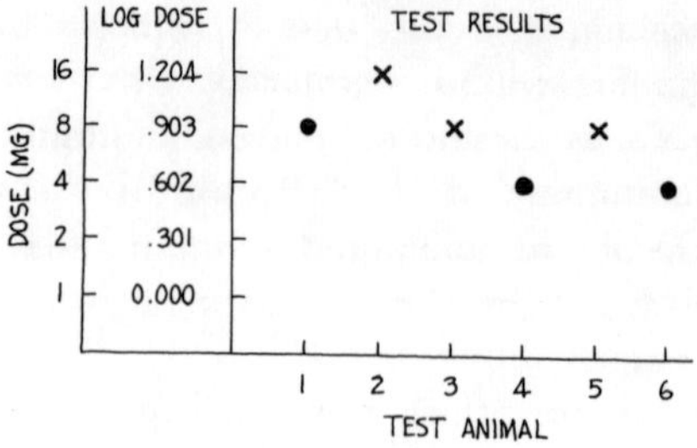

FIGURE 2

Results of a sequence of six tests using the up-and-down method

as possible, and since our supply of scorpion fish venom is limited we must try to get a good estimate from a small number of tests.

One design that has good properties is conducted one test at a time and consists of merely increasing the dose for the next animal if the last one tested did not respond to the dose administered and of decreasing the dose if the last animal did respond.

Let us examine the up-and-down version of our scorpion fish venom experiment in detail, limiting ourselves, for brevity, to animals of the same weight and a fixed venom concentration. For a particular concentration and animal weight, we proceed to test several animals at different dosages following our planned strategy.

We prepare to administer doses of sizes 1, 2, 4, 8, and 16 mg, and we begin by testing the first animal at any one of these levels. We choose, say, 8 mg for the first dose; the animal survives, and we record an O toward the left in Figure 2. The next animal is given the next higher dose of 16 mg. It does not survive; nor does the third animal (tested at 8 mg). In all, six animals are tested following this rule. From the data of Figure 2, because none of the 4 mg and two-thirds of the 8 mg doses produced a response, we might guess that the average threshold is somewhere between 4 mg and 8 mg. We would be uncertain, and we would not have a systematic way of making an estimate. A fairly precise estimate can be obtained, however, by averaging the levels at which the tests were done (in logarithmic units). Greater precision can be obtained by using a special table worked out mathematically to obtain the best estimate possible. By using this strategy, we can obtain about as much information from six animals as we could obtain by testing 20 animals in the design of Table 1 and Figure 1. The sequential character of the new approach tends to concentrate the doses where they are needed to get a good estimate.

The technique is also one of extreme simplicity to use. The sequence of trials in Figure 2 is completely described by indicating the sequence of O's and X's as they are observed and stating the dosage interval and the dosage administered on the last trial. For the example in Figure 2, the series is OXXOXO; the spacing of doses is log 2 = .301, and the final test dose was 4, which, in logarithmic units, is log 4 = .602. The average threshold dosage is estimated to be

$$.602 + k(.301)$$

where a value for k may be obtained from a table in Dixon and Massey (1969) for the configuration OXXOXO. The value of k is .831, so the estimate is

$$.602 + .831(.301) = .852$$

Because .852 is the logarithm of 7.11 we obtain 7.11 mg for our estimate of the average threshold dose.

SUMMARY

We have illustrated the solution to a measurement or assay problem in which a special design of the sequence to be followed in the collection of the data allows us to get the resulting estimate with high efficiency. Other results of the statistical theory forming the basis of this procedure also show that this is about as good as we can do when we are able to observe only whether we exceed or fall short of the desired level. The theory shows that it requires only twice as many observations to obtain a threshold estimate of the same accuracy as would be obtained if we could measure precisely the exact dosage corresponding to each animal's own threshold. This, of course, is an impossibility for poisons, although we can imagine coming close to it in some problem where repeated measurements of the same animal are possible.

PROBLEMS

1. Give three examples (not mentioned in the article) where appraising strength of material is needed.

2. In the 7th sentence of the example of appraising scorpion fish venom, explain the meaning of the words "on the average."

3. What is the threshold level of an animal?

4. How does this article define the average threshold level for the scorpion fish venom experiment? Would you use the same criterion to

define the threshold level when deciding the dosage level of curare to be used in medical procedures with human beings?

5. What are the advantages of a sequential testing procedure?

6. In Figure 2 we notice that the 1st animal survived when administered a dose of 8 mg. and the 2nd animal died when administered 16 mg. Why don't we conclude at this point that the threshold is between 8 and 16 mg.?

7. In the sequential up-and-down method of finding a dosage level, when does one stop taking samples?

8. Suppose we test 7 animals at the 5 dosage levels of venom described in the text, and obtain the series of responses XXOXOOX, with the final test dose being 8. Draw the results of the sequence of 7 tests similar to Figure 2. Estimate the average threshold, using the value $k = -1.237$ obtained from Dixon and Massey (1969).

9. Draw a graph similar to Figure 2 for the punch example. (Hint: use "parts of gin" as dosage level.) Can you estimate the average desired strength of punch by the up-and-down method described later in the text? Why or why not?

REFERENCES

J. J. Blum, R. Crease, D. J. Jenden, and N. W. Scholes. 1957. "The Mechanism of Action of Ryanodine on Skeletal Muscle." *Journal of Pharmacology and Experimental Therapeutics* 111:477–486.

Lincoln P. Brower, William N. Ryerson, Lorna L. Coppinger, and Susan C. Glazier. 1968. "Ecological Chemistry and the Palatability Spectrum." *Science* 161:1349–1351.

W. J. Dixon and F. J. Massey, Jr. 1969. *Introduction to Statistical Analysis,* Third Edition. New York: McGraw-Hill.

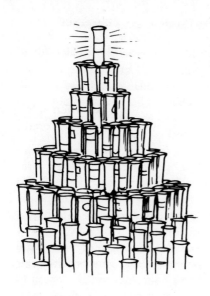

DRUG SCREENING: The Never-Ending Search for New and Better Drugs

Charles W. Dunnett   *Lederle Laboratories Division, American Cyanamid Company*

PROBABLY EVERYONE can recall reading about a small boat lost at sea or an aircraft down in some unpopulated area involving a search for survivors. If the search is successful, both rescuers and rescued receive wide public acclaim. On the other hand, if the search is unsuccessful, the episode is soon forgotten. In neither case do we see much in the press about the planning and organization of the search. We can imagine, however, what a tremendous effort it must be to map out the area to be explored, to marshal the needed resources in aircraft and other vehicles, and to use all the available people and equipment so as to maximize the chance of a successful outcome in the shortest possible time.

Pharmaceutical companies conduct somewhat similar searches for new drugs, but their search is continuous. Just as a rescue team has some idea where to look, perhaps based on a radio message received from the victims, so research chemists often know what types of chemical structures to look for to treat a particular disease, and the chemists can set about synthesizing compounds of the desired type. Sometimes, however, their knowledge may be vague, resulting in such a wide range of possibilities that many, many compounds have to be made and tested. In such a case, the search is very lengthy and requires years of effort by many people to develop a useful new drug.

Researching thousands of compounds for the few that might be effective requires highly organized, efficient testing methods. With an inefficient procedure, progress will be slow and the testing laboratory may never get to the "good" compounds. Of course, the procedure used to test each compound must have a high degree of accuracy and must be capable of detecting a good compound.

Testing a long series of compounds in the search for any that have useful biological properties is known as *drug screening*. Drug screening requires laboratories, technical personnel to operate them, and appropriate apparatus and instruments. Ordinarily, laboratory tests are conducted with animals, which must be housed, cared for, and observed in the laboratory. Space limitations together with the limitations of the staff severely restrict the number of compounds that can be assessed. A single laboratory cannot hope to test more than several hundred, or, perhaps, a few thousand, compounds annually for a specified biological activity. This testing rate cannot even keep up with the rate of synthesis of new compounds. Yet, if all the laboratories throughout the entire pharmaceutical industry are considered, much is accomplished. It is estimated (Arnow 1970), for example, that approximately 175,000 substances are subjected to biologic evaluation each year.

The screening test is only the first hurdle along the path of developing an effective drug; much further testing and investigation needs to be done before the drug can be tried on humans. In fact, only about 20 of the 175,000 substances tested finally become available in the local drug store.

Anything that improves the efficiency of the testing procedure increases the chance of discovering a new cure. Naturally, the biologist designing a new screening procedure attempts to use an animal and test system that reflect the human disease for which a cure is being sought as accurately as possible and yet are easy to use in the laboratory. We will not deal with this aspect of the problem here, but rather with the contribution of statistics to improvement of drug screening procedures.

AN EXAMPLE: ANTICANCER SCREENING

In drug screening, the animals of a sample treated with a particular compound are observed to determine whether the treatment is having a desirable effect. Perhaps all that is noted in each animal is whether or not it is "cured" or shows improvement. The result of the test can be expressed simply as the number of cured or improved animals out of the total number tested. Since not every animal responds to treatment in exactly the same way, the number cured might be 0, 1, 2, or all the way up to the whole sample size.

More often, a measurement of some sort is made upon each animal, the magnitude being indicative of the treatment effect. For example, in anti-cancer screening, after implanting cancer cells in mice, the investigator treats them with the test chemical compound to see whether it retards the growth of the cancer tumors. After treating the mice for a fixed length of time, he removes the tumors and weighs them. For comparison, a similar group of untreated "control" animals is handled in the same way except for the absence of the chemical treatment. If the chemical is effective, the tumor weights of the treated mice should be less than the tumor weights of the control mice. The statistician's job is to help decide, on the basis of the numerical values obtained, whether the tested compound merits further investigation.

The following are actual tumor weights observed in three animals treated with a test compound and in six untreated control animals:

Treated: 0.96, 1.59, 1.14 grams
Controls: 1.29, 1.60, 2.27, 1.31, 1.88, 2.21 grams

The reason for having more control animals than treated is that, in one experiment perhaps 30 to 40 different compounds will be tested, each one in a different set of three animals. One control group suffices, however, to compare with the results from all the test compounds; hence it is desirable to have it larger in size in order to obtain a more precise control average.

Note the high variability from one animal to another. This is typical of the biological variation in screening tests that makes it difficult to determine with certainty whether the treated animals have really improved as a result of the treatment. How might a statistician go about deciding whether a compound has any merit?

DRUG SCREENING AS A DECISION PROBLEM

In drug screening, two actions are possible: (1) to "reject" the drug, meaning to conclude that the tested drug has little or no effect, in which case it will be set aside and a new drug selected for screening, and (2) to "accept" the drug provisionally, in which case it will be subjected to further, more refined experimentation.

To abandon a drug when in fact it is a useful one (a *false negative*) is clearly undesirable, yet there is always some risk of that. On the other hand, to go ahead with further, more expensive testing of a drug that is in fact useless (a *false positive*) wastes time and money that could have been spent on testing other compounds. .

Thus, we are faced with what is known in statistics as a *decision problem:* how to use available experimental data to choose between alternative courses of action in a rational way.

AN APPROACH TO SOLVING THE PROBLEM

What would the drug screening investigator like to achieve? A virtually unlimited supply of compounds is available for testing, more than he can hope to test over any reasonable period of time. Most of them lack the biological activity he is searching for, but (hopefully) a few of them possess it. His goal is to find as many of these active compounds as possible with the facilities at his disposal.

As a hypothetical, but not entirely unrealistic, example, let us suppose there are 10,000 compounds of which 40 are active and the remaining 9960 are inactive. The investigator is screening the drugs for antitumor activity, and he tests them by treating groups of three tumor-bearing mice with each compound, comparing the resulting tumor weights with the corresponding values for six control animals observed in the same experiment. He wishes to accept or reject each test compound on the basis of the observed tumor weights. Typically, about 50 compounds per week can be tested in this way, so that about four years' work will be required for all 10,000 compounds. Over this period of time, it is inevitable that some of the 9960 inactive compounds submitted to the screening will pass. The follow-up tests required on these false positives will require test facilities that could have been employed to screen some new compounds. Often the next step after a compound passes the screening step is to carry out a "dose-response" study, which consists of treating groups of animals with several dose levels of a drug in order to determine the relationship between dose and response. At this step, the inactive false positive compounds generally will be eliminated. Suppose, for illustration, that 30 animals are required for each compound at this step. This means that to follow up each compound accepted by the screening, it will be necessary to forgo or postpone the testing of ten new compounds.

Consider the experimental data given above. The mean, or average, tumor weight for the treated animals is $(0.96 + 1.59 + 1.14)/3 = 1.23$ grams. Comparing this with the corresponding mean for the six control animals, $(1.29 + 1.60 + 2.27 + 1.31 + 1.88 + 2.21)/6 = 1.76$ grams, we see that a reduction of $1.76 - 1.23 = 0.53$ gram has apparently been obtained. If the drug has no effect, a zero reduction would be "expected," but, of course, the variability of the animals makes it likely that some difference between the two means would occur even if the drug has no effect Thus, the researcher must decide how large a difference he requires the drug to show before he decides to "accept" it.

Let us assume for the moment that a reduction of 0.53 gram in tumor weight is not enough to convince our investigator that the compound is an active one; let's say that he requires a reduction of 0.70 gram before he will permit the compound to pass the screening test. What are the consequences of setting a cut-off value of 0.70 gram in screening the 10,000 compounds?

What he really needs to know is how many of the 9960 inactive compounds and 40 active compounds will pass the test. He could go ahead and screen the compounds using the 0.70-gram criterion, but it would take several years to collect the results: this would be rather late to find out that he made an unwise choice in the cut-off criterion.

Fortunately, there is another way to get at this problem. Statisticians have a unit, or yardstick, called the *standard error*, which they use to determine how often measures like the difference between two means will exceed any specified limit. An estimate of the standard error needed in our case could be calculated from the observed data, but it would be unreliable because of the small number of observations. It is possible, however, to estimate the standard error accurately from other data of the same type, which, in routine screening, are available in large quantities from past records. Suppose that, for tumor weights, the standard error of a difference between a mean of six control tumor weights and a mean of three treated tumor weights is known to be 0.35 gram.

The next step is to divide the difference between the cut-off value and the *expected* value of the test statistic by this standard error. For an inactive compound, our researcher would expect the two mean tumor weights to be the same; hence the test statistic is expected to have the value zero. The cut-off value of 0.70 gram, therefore, is $(0.70 - 0)/0.35 = 2.0$ standard errors from the zero expectation. Consulting a table of the *normal distribution* (available in most statistics texts) he finds that a deviation of 2.0 or more standard errors from the expected value occurs with a probability of .0228. This means that he can expect to observe a misleading reduction in tumor weight exceeding 0.7 gram for approximately 23 out of 1000 inactive drugs submitted to screening. In other words, of the 9960 inactive compounds, $.0228 \times 9960 = 227$ of them can be expected to pass as false positives.

Consider next the 40 active compounds: how many of them can be expected to pass? This is a more difficult question, because the answer depends on how active they really are. It is not to be expected that even a very active compound will eliminate the tumor completely in the relatively short time the animals are under treatment. Modest decreases in tumor size are the most that researchers can hope for.

Let us assume for now, rather arbitrarily, that the 40 active compounds are each capable of reducing tumor weight by 0.7 gram (the same as that required by our cut-off criterion). As each active compound is tested, some actually will result in a reduction of more than 0.7 gram, while others will give rise to smaller reductions, because of the inevitable variability of the animals. Therefore, only half of the actives can be expected to show a reduction exceeding the stipulated cut-off value and, hence, to pass the test.

This means that on the average, the accepted compounds will consist of 20 actives (true positives) and 227 false positives. The follow-up testing required on each is the equivalent of ten screening tests, so, in addition to the 10,000 screening tests, there will be $247 \times 10 = 2470$ follow-up tests, or 12,470 tests in all. For this effort, the researcher can expect to find 20 active compounds under the assumptions about the composition of the original set of 10,000 compounds and the degree of activity of the actives. It is useful to express this as a "yield" per thousand tests. Using 0.7 gram as the cut-off value, the resulting yield is

$$\frac{20}{12,470} \times 1000 = 1.60 \text{ actives/thousand tests.}$$

Next, consider the consequences of altering the criterion for a compound to pass the screen. Suppose that instead of a 0.7 gram reduction in tumor weight, a cut-off value of 0.6 gram is used. This corresponds to a **deviation** of $0.6/0.35 = 1.71$ on the normal curve, and the corresponding probability obtained from tables of the normal distribution is .0436. Thus, of the inactive compounds tested, $.0436 \times 9960 = 434$ false positives are expected to occur.

What about the 40 active compounds? The researcher still assumes that each has a degree of activity capable of producing a reduction of 0.7 gram on the average. How many of them will actually produce a reduction of 0.6 gram or more? Expressing the difference of 0.1 gram as a deviation on the normal curve by dividing by the standard error, he obtains $0.1/0.35 = 0.29$; from the normal tables, he finds that the corresponding probability is .6140. Hence, using 0.6 gram as the passing criterion, he can expect $.6140 \times 40 = 25$ active compounds to pass. This results in $434 + 25 = 459$ compounds passing the screen, so the total testing effort is now $10,000 + 459 \times 10 = 14,590$ tests. Thus the yield per thousand tests is

$$\frac{25}{14,590} \times 1000 = 1.71 \text{ actives/thousand tests,}$$

an increase of 0.11 over the yield obtained using 0.7 gram as the cut-off value.

Now it should be clear how to go about "optimizing" the choice of the cut-off value for the given hypothetical structure of the compounds. It is necessary to try various cut-off values to determine the yield for each in the above way. Figure 1 shows a curve of the computed yield plotted against

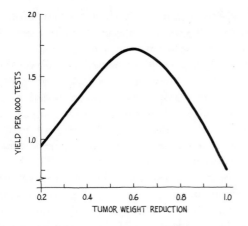

FIGURE 1

Yields for one-stage screening tests

the corresponding cut-off value. It can be seen that the point of maximum yield is easily determined and, in fact, occurs very close to a cut-off value of 0.6 gram reduction. Of course, this applies only to the particular hypothetical mix of active and inactive compounds that we have assumed; we will come back to this point later. For this particular mix, a yield of 1.71 per thousand tests appears to be about the best that can be obtained.

SEQUENTIAL PROCEDURES FOR DRUG SCREENING

It is possible, however, to do still better by using another type of screening. Statistical theory tells us that a kind of test procedure, known as a *sequential test,* is more efficient for reaching decisions of the type we need. In sequential testing, the number of tests is not fixed in advance; rather, the testing proceeds sequentially and the number of tests depends upon the results observed. This gives us the option, after observing a test result on a compound, to forgo making an immediate decision about that compound and to subject the compound to another test. From the results of a second test averaged with those of a first test, we may conclude that further testing is unnecessary, or we may forgo a decision again and wait for a third test result on the compound. This process could go on until a decision is reached to accept or reject the compound. Of course, if too many stages are permitted, the procedure loses efficiency because of the delay and because of the extra trouble involved in keeping a sufficient supply of the compound on hand to repeat the test. In drug screening applications, it has usually been found best to limit the testing to two or three stages.

A sequential procedure is more efficient because it allows us to compile additional data on the compounds about which doubt exists, without much increase in the average amount of testing required, because additional testing needs to be done only on a relatively few compounds.

Suppose that we decide to reject a compound without further testing if a tumor weight reduction of less than 0.2 gram is observed on the first test. If, instead, a reduction of more than 0.2 gram is obtained, we will test the compound again on another group of mice. At the end of this second stage of testing, the tumor weight reduction will be measured as usual, and its value will be averaged with the value obtained for that compound in the first stage. If the average of these two values exceeds 0.5 gram, we will accept the compound; otherwise it will be discarded. For obvious reasons, a procedure of this type is called a *two-stage test* (the procedure discussed in the previous section is called a *one-stage test*).

For illustration, consider our numerical example. For that set of data, the observed tumor weight reduction turned out to be 0.53 gram. Using a one-stage test, we found that the optimum cut-off value was 0.6 gram, which would require this compound to be discarded. With the two-stage test described in the preceding paragraph, however, it would be tested again. Suppose another test (using three treated and six control animals) gave a tumor weight reduction of 0.49 gram. Averaging the two results, 0.53 and 0.49, we obtain 0.51 gram; this is enough for the compound to be accepted.

What are the consequences of using the two-stage test on the hypothetical mix of 10,000 active and inactive compounds? First of all, the amount of testing obviously will be increased because, for some compounds, two tests will have to be run. The amount of increase can be computed. For an inactive compound, the probability of obtaining a tumor weight reduction in excess of 0.2 gram turns out to be .284. Thus, $.284 \times 9960 = 2829$ of the inactive compounds will require two screening tests to permit a decision, the remainder requiring only one test. For an active compound, the corresponding probability is .923; hence, $.923 \times 40 = 37$ of the actives will be tested a second time. Therefore, the total number of screening tests required to screen the 10,000 compounds is $10,000 + 2829 + 37 = 12,866$ (compared to 10,000 in a one-stage procedure).

It is also fairly easy to work out the probability that an inactive compound passes the screening under the sequential procedure; this may be done for an active compound as well. For an active compound, the probability is .77; thus, $.77 \times 40 = 31$ active compounds can be expected to pass. For an inactive compound, the probability is .020; hence, $.020 \times 9960 = 199$ false positives will occur. Therefore, a total of 230 compounds are expected to pass, entailing an additional testing effort equal to 2300 tests. This makes altogether $12,866 + 2300 = 15,166$ tests. The yield per thousand tests for this scheme is

$$\frac{31}{15,166} \times 1000 = 2.04 \text{ actives/thousand tests};$$

note that this is higher than the best yield that can be obtained with a one-stage test.

By trying various cut-off values for the two stages of the test, an optimum two-stage screening test can be devised. The optimum yield turns out to be 2.15 per thousand tests, achieved with a cut-off value of 0.4 gram reduction at the first stage and 0.5 gram reduction at the second stage. The increase in yield from 1.71 per thousand with the best one-stage test to 2.15 per thousand using the best two-stage test represents an improvement of 26% in the efficiency of the screening test. This is an important advance because it means that useful cures for diseases can be found more quickly.

Further improvements can be obtained by considering more than two stages of testing. We will not go into the details here, but an optimum three-stage test can be devised to yield 2.33 per thousand. More than three stages can be considered, but it is questionable whether the increases in efficiency that theoretically could be obtained are worth the extra complication. (Complicated bookkeeping in a large laboratory has its own high costs in both potential errors and manpower.)

EFFECT OF ASSUMPTION ABOUT THE COMPOSITION OF THE COMPOUNDS BEING SCREENED

In the forgoing we showed how the statistician can optimize the choice of the cut-off values that determine whether a given compound should be accepted, rejected, or tested again. The optimum, however, was based on a hypothetical mixture of active and inactive compounds being screened. We assumed that 10,000 compounds contained 9960 inactives and 40 actives; moreover, we assumed the active compounds had a degree of activity capable of reducing the animal tumor weights by 0.7 gram.

Of course, the statistician must repeat the whole process for other assumptions about the composition of the compounds being screened to determine the effects on the optimum cut-off values. It turns out that the actual *number* of actives assumed to be in the mix does not affect the screening procedure. In other words, if the 10,000 compounds contained 100 actives, or 4 actives, or only 1, instead of 40, the same screening criteria would produce an optimum yield. (Of course, the actual *magnitude* of the optimum yield would go up or down with the number of actives assumed to be present.) On the other hand, the degree of activity assumed for the active compounds does affect the procedure. All the statistician can do here is to work out the best procedure for various degrees of activity and let the screening investigator decide on the basis of his knowledge what level of activity of interest to him is most likely to occur. Then the statistician can tell him what screening criteria will produce the optimum results for that level of activity. It is also possible to consider a mixture of two, three, or even several different levels of activity among the active compounds.

OTHER VARIABLES IN THE SCREENING PROCEDURE

In the preceding discussion, it was assumed that the test procedure itself was fixed and the only variables were the cut-off criteria. Other factors, however, also can be altered, for example, the number of animals used in each test. Is the choice of three animals for each test compound and six animals for control really best? A reduction in either of these numbers would enable the investigator to test more compounds in each experiment. On the debit side, however, this would increase the standard error of the test statistic, which would have the undesirable effect of increasing the chances for a compound to be misclassified.

The statistician can study the effect of changes in these variables on the theoretical yield, by carrying out calculations similar to those we have already described. The object is to achieve, with the test facilities that are available, the greatest expected yield in terms of active compounds found. Of course, it is impossible to guarantee what results will actually be obtained. No matter how efficient a screening procedure is, in fact, there may be *no* active compounds presented for screening. In the end, we must depend upon the ingenuity of the chemists to produce compounds that have the desired activity.

APPLICATIONS

Statistical studies of the sort described here have improved the efficiency of many of the routine screening procedures in our laboratories. The anticancer screening program is discussed in detail by Vogel and Haynes (1962), who state that an increase in the screening rate from 450 compounds per year to 1300 per year has been achieved. I could provide a happy ending to this tale if I could tell you about the discovery of a new cure for cancer as a result, but although some possible leads have been discovered, it seems that we are still a very long way from this goal. Past successes in other areas, such as the remarkable discovery of the antibiotic Aureomycin after the screening of over 4000 soil samples, are convincing proof, however, that drug screening plays a necessary and important role in the never-ending search for new and better drugs. A recent book by Arnow (1970) contains an interesting account of this and other aspects of drug research.

The statistical aspects of drug screening are similar to screening and selection problems in other fields. For example, in the development of new and improved strains of an agricultural crop, such as wheat, each potential new strain must be planted and grown, and measurements of its yield and other indicators of performance must be taken. On the basis of the results, some strains are chosen to be planted again on a wider scale, and eventually, after many repetitions of the cycle, a new variety may emerge to replace current standard varieties. The plant breeder, like the drug screener, must determine how best to use his facilities for testing various candidates in order to maximize the chances of success. My 1968 article gives a more general discussion of the problems of screening and selection.

PROBLEMS

1. Why are there more control animals than treated animals in the anticancer screening example?

2. What are the two actions possible in the drug screening experiment viewed as a decision problem?

3. Explain what this article means by "false negative" and "false positive."

4. If a cut-off value of .8 gm. is used in the anticancer screening example then from tables of the normal distribution, one finds that .0107 of the inactive compounds are expected to be false positives and .3859 of the active compounds to pass. Using the above information calculate the yield per thousand tests in a one-stage testing procedure. Compare with the value obtained from Figure 1.

5. Suppose that two different laboratories were to screen the same 10,000 compounds using the same screening procedure. Would they necessarily obtain the same number of active compounds? Would they necessarily obtain the same active compounds if they obtained the same number of compounds? Why or why not?

6. In a real experiment the number of active compounds among the total number of compounds tested is unknown. How would a statistician go about deciding the optimal cut-off point?

7. Define a "two-stage test" and a "one-stage test." State the advantages and disadvantages of each type of test.

8. What would be the yield of active compounds per 1000 tests if the investigator requires an average reduction of .80 grams in tumor weight before he will permit the compound to pass the screening test? Can you find a different reduction that gives the same yield? Which of the two would you prefer? (Use Figure 1.)

REFERENCES

L. E. Arnow. 1970. *Health in a Bottle; Searching for the Drugs that Help.* Philadelphia: Lippincott.

C. W. Dunnett. 1968. "Screening and Selection." D. L. Sills, ed., *International Encyclopedia of the Social Sciences* vol. 14. New York: Macmillan and Free Press.

A. W. Vogel and J. D. Haynes. 1962. "Experiences with Sequential Screening for Anticancer Agents." *Cancer Chemotherapy Reports* 22:23–30.

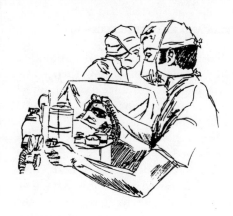

HOW FREQUENTLY DO INNOVATIONS
SUCCEED IN SURGERY AND ANESTHESIA?

John P. Gilbert   *Harvard University*
Bucknam McPeek   *Massachusetts General Hospital, Boston*
Frederick Mosteller   *Harvard University*

WHEN THERAPIES are compared for effectiveness, what happens? How often does an innovation appear to be superior to its competitors? When innovations are successful, for example, the Salk vaccine or the development of successful organ transplantation, society gains a major victory. This paper studies the effectiveness of new surgical and anesthetic therapies in their clinical setting.

We reviewed a sample of 107 published papers appraising surgical and anesthetic treatments. Of these therapies sufficiently promising to be tested in human patients, we ask what proportion have proved to be substantial improvements over existing ones? What proportion have been moderately successful? And what proportion have been found to be less effective than had been hoped and expected?

Using these papers, we assess the percentage improvement a new innovation is apt to make, as well as the chance that it will turn out to have been an improvement at all. Thus our aim is to describe the crop of newly tested therapies for effectiveness compared with that of the treatments they are designed to replace.

Except for a major breakthrough like the introduction of antibiotics, we have little reason to suppose that the development of new therapeutic ideas will change drastically. Thus, we assume that a similar distribution of successes and failures will occur in the near future. The results presented here should give realistic expectations at least for the short term.

We drew a sample of papers evaluating different treatments actually given to patients. To get this sample, we turned to the National Library of Medicine's MEDical Literature Analysis and Retrieval System (MEDLARS). Computer-produced bibliographies can be retrieved from this data base which, since January 1964, has provided an exhaustive coverage of the world's medical literature. By searching the system for prospective studies (see the essay by Brown) of specified surgical operations or anesthetic drugs, we were able to gather papers whose authors used human patients to evaluate surgical and anesthetic treatments. The papers appeared between 1964 and 1972.

We considered only papers in English because of our own language disabilities, and papers with ten or more patients in a group because we wanted to study large investigations rather than case studies. Any other bias in the sample selections, then, arose from peculiarities of the MEDLARS indexing system and contents at the time of the search rather than from our prejudices.

The papers included many kinds of studies. To give an idea of the variety, some dealt with ulcers, appendectomy, cirrhosis, cancers, bone operations, colon operations, major vascular operations, stab wounds, antibiotics, clot prevention, drainage, and the impact of anesthetic drugs and techniques.

Our sampled papers reported on three basic types of studies—*randomized controlled trials, non-randomized controlled trials,* and *series.* We use the term randomized controlled trials when the investigator compared two or more treatment groups and assigned patients to the groups by a formal randomization process (such as drawing random numbers to decide which treatment is assigned to each patient). The non-randomized controlled trials did not have such a formal randomization process and varied from comparing groups treated concurrently in the same institution to comparing patients treated previously by one method with patients treated currently with another. The papers reporting on series described sets of patients treated in some specified manner but with no comparison except possibly with other reports in the literature dealing with similar patients. In the rest of this paper we are concerned with only the papers dealing with randomized controlled trials.

If our MEDLARS approach were perfect and produced all the papers, one might think that we have a census rather than a sample of papers. To adopt this attitude would be to misunderstand our purpose. We think of a process producing these research studies through time, and we think of our sample—even if it were a census—as a sample in time from this continuing process. Thus our inference would be to the general process, even if we did have all appropriate papers from a time period.

In appraising the results of comparative investigations, we take several simplifying actions.

First, we classify each therapy as either an *innovation* or as a *standard*. Some diseases have a widely recognized standard therapy against which all others are measured. A good example of this has been (the standard) radical mastectomy for cancer of the breast. In such instances the standard is easy to recognize; all others can be considered as competing innovations regardless of how recent their introduction. We have used the letter "I" to denote the treatment we regarded as an innovation and the letter "S" for the standard.

Ideally one wishes an analysis to produce the maximum amount of information contained in a body of data. It is often impractical to achieve this in practice. Thus in trying to evaluate the difference in performance between standard programs and innovations in our study we were unable to assign a highly accurate and precise value to the observed differences. In many studies we are content with knowing how many differences were positive and how many negative. In our data often the two programs were essentially equal in performance and so it was useful to acknowledge this in the scale. In addition sometimes one program was not only better but was clearly much better, and it was not hard to make a distinction between these two. The five point scale that we have used is a happy solution to this problem because it is relatively simple and easy to apply and it retains most of the relevant information that we need. The five point scale is widely used in both social science and medicine because it allows us to capture much of the information we want in a practical manner.

Second, we speak below of a pair of competitive therapies as having three possible relations: About equal (S=I), the first named preferred to the second named (S>I or I>S), and the first named *highly* preferred to the second named (S>>I or I>>S). We have tried to report on this scale what we think the original investigators would have reported. Usually their words make this clear.

Third, we have divided therapies into two classes: *Primary* therapies intended to cure or ameliorate the patient's primary disease, and *secondary* therapies intended to prevent or treat such complications as infection or thromboembolic disease or to offer improvements in anesthesia or postoperative care. The basic 107 studies included 36 randomized clinical trials. Of these 36 papers, 21 deal with *primary* therapies and 15 deal with *secondary* therapies. For technical reasons* several studies had to be set aside, also

---

*One study had too many comparisons; another had too small a sample size for its complicated design.

some studies had more than one comparison. In Table I, we deal with comparisons, rather than studies. By coincidence the number of papers equals the number of comparisons in the analysis.

Referring to Table 1 for randomized trials, we see that in five of the 36 comparisons, or about 14%, an innovation was highly preferred to a standard. In 16 comparisons, including the previous five, about 44%, the new therapy was regarded as successful, sometimes because it was no worse than a standard and thus became available as an alternative.

TABLE 1.   Summary for Innovations in Randomized Clinical Trials

		PRIMARY	SECONDARY	TOTAL
I > > S:	Innovation highly preferred	1	4	5
I > S:	Innovation preferred	5	2	7
I = S:	About equal, innovation a success	2	2	4
I = S:	About equal, innovation a disappointment	7	3	10
S > I:	Standard preferred	3	3	6
S > > I:	Standard highly preferred	1	3	4
	Comparisons	19	17	36

In 10, or 28%, the equality of an innovation with a standard could be regarded as a disappointment because, although the innovation was more trouble or more costly or more risky, it did not perform better. In 20 comparisons, about 56%, a standard was preferred (counting innovative disappointments) to an innovation.

Overall, Table 1 shows that innovations highly preferred to standard treatments are hard but not impossible to find, and that almost half of the innovations provided some positive gain. It is worth reflecting on what our attitude might be toward extreme findings in either direction. Suppose that nearly all studies, or even the lion's share, found the innovation highly preferred; one would have to conclude that standard therapies were fairly easy to improve on and indeed that the kind of medicine being appraised was in its infancy or else that a sudden breakthrough had been made on all fronts. This is unlikely with as many different diseases and therapies as occur in the sample. At another extreme, if no substantial gains occurred, the suggestion is that the field has topped out, at least during the period of the study, awaiting some new insights.

Figure 1 summarizes 11 primary studies in which survival was an appropriate measure of outcome and plots the percentage of survivors, often after many years, for the standard therapy against that for the innovation. Two papers had two comparisons of a standard against an innovation, making 13 comparisons in all. The seven points below the 45° diagonal line show the

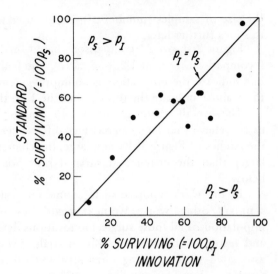

FIGURE 1

Primary Therapies—Survival Percentages

Points falling below the 45° line indicate higher survival rates for the innovation than for the standard. Primary therapies are intended to cure the patient's disease.

innovation performing better; the six points above show the standard performing better. The greatest observed gain (shown by the point farthest below the line with coordinates (74%, 49%)) comes from a study of therapeutic portacaval shunt. Curiously, the point farthest above the line (showing the greatest apparent loss) corresponds to a study of the same operation performed prophylactically, in advance of urgent need (32%, 50%). The overall impression given by the figure is one of points rather closely hugging the diagonal line. The degree of scatter from the line depends in part upon

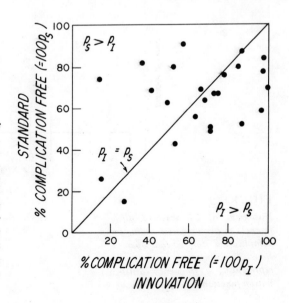

FIGURE 2

Secondary Therapies—Percentage Free of Complication

Percentages avoiding specific post-operative complications. Secondary therapies are intended to reduce the frequency of post-operative complications. Points below the 45° line indicate fewer complications of a specific sort accompanying the innovation than the standard. The innovations have 15 below, 8 above, and 1 on the line.

the size of samples (number of patients used in the studies), and we explore this idea further later.

Figure 2 shows 24 comparisons based on 11 secondary studies (five had 1 comparison, four had 2, one had 3, one had 8). The 15 points below the line indicate the innovation as an improvement over the standard treatment; the 8 above indicate the reverse, and the 1 on the line gives a tie.

The overall scatter about the 45° line in Figure 2 is large, encouraging us to believe that larger percentage differences have been found here than in the studies of Figure 1. By and large, the changes in rate of complications are larger than the changes in survival rate. We make this more quantitative below.

In the work reported so far, some innovations performed better than a standard, others worse. We next regard these outcomes as a sample from the population of all those surgical innovations developed by our medical system and tested by randomized clinical trials. Every study has its uncertainties associated with sampling variability and other sources of unreliability. We want to allow for sampling variability in our description of the gains and losses. The general idea is that if we focus on a particular sort of performance, we may be able to gather strength from several studies even though they deal with disparate operations. For example, among the primary studies we focus on those where the main hope from the operation is the extension of life. Then we might ask about the distribution (variety) of improvements actually achieved by this type of innovation.

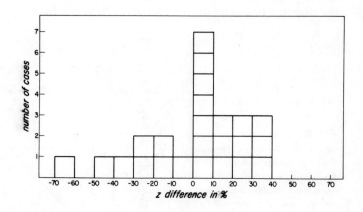

FIGURE 3

Histogram of 24 observed differences in percentages avoiding a complication for several operations. This illustrates one way of representing a frequency distribution function.

We use the idea of distributions, and so we want to illustrate what these are. In our study of post-operative complications we had 24 differences of the form: the percentage of patients who did not develop complication under the innovation MINUS the percentage who did not develop the complication under the standard. We use these 24 differences for illustration. We can ask of the data how many differences were in intervals of length 10 such as between 0 and 9%, 10% and 19%, or between –20% and –29%. This information is presented graphically in Figure 3.

Seven of the differences fell in the interval 0 to 9%, three in each of the intervals 10 to 19%, 20 to 29%, and 30 to 39%, while one was so low that it fell in the interval –60% to –70%. Thus Figure 3 gives us an idea of how these differences are distributed with regard to their values. If we had had many values we could have made much smaller intervals and we could think of it being very like an idealized smooth curve that might look like:

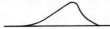

This curve is called the density function of the distribution.

Often it is more relevant or convenient to ask how many data points were larger than a particular value on the scale, rather than asking how many data points were within a particular interval as we did above. If we represent this way of looking at the data graphically we obtain Figure 4.

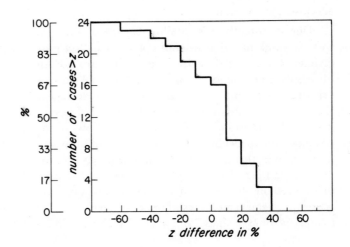

FIGURE 4

Frequency distribution cumulated from the right to show the frequency of getting a given percent difference at least as large as the one on the horizontal axis.

Figure 4 was obtained by adding up the number of squares, i.e. observations, to the right of each point on the horizontal scale of Figure 1. For this reason it is called a cumulative distribution function. If again we think of having many more points and using much smaller intervals we might find the figure to approach a continuous curve that is the cumulative distribution function that corresponds to the continuous density pictured above. This curve looks like:

%
100

0

difference

When the vertical axis is a percent or a proportion, we can read off the estimated probability of a difference at least as large as the one on the horizontal axis.

If every study were based on an enormous sample of patients, so that sampling errors would be very small, the reports of gains and losses would give us the distribution of differences in true performance between innovations and standards in our sample of papers. In turn that sample distribution would estimate the distribution of gains in the population—the process generating these studies and comparisons. But studies are of necessity limited in size, and, in reports of small studies, differences vary more due to sampling error than in large ones. We need to have a way to pool the results of such studies, large and small, that will give an idea of the distribution of *true* gains and losses in the trials.

One such method is to allow for the sampling variability associated with specific randomized trials and come up with a pooled figure. The observed difference may be thought of as having two additive components—the true difference plus the sampling error. A special statistical technique called analysis of variance produces estimates of the average and standard deviation of the sample of true differences. (The standard deviation measures how spread out the distribution is.) We can estimate how often various sizes of gains can be expected to occur by making an assumption about the true differences, namely that the differences approximately follow a normal distribution. (The word normal here applies to a particular shape of distribution—it is not being used in the sense of normal versus abnormal. Heights of adults and scores on achievement tests are examples of distributions that are approximately normal in shape. A normal distribution looks something like

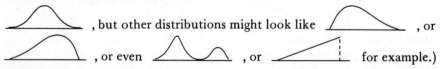

, but other distributions might look like   , or   , or even   , or   for example.)

It is important to understand that this method develops summary statistics for *true* gains and losses *across* studies. The statistics reported are (a) the estimated average true gain, averaged across comparisons, and (b) the estimated standard deviation of the true gain, averaged across comparisons. If, for example, the average gain were 0% and the standard deviation of the gain 6%, our assumption of a normal distribution allows us to calculate that gains of 10% or more could occur in about one-twentieth of the opportunities. It would still be true that the gain would be positive for about half the innovations and negative (that is, a loss) in half, in agreement with Table 1. It then becomes the goal of clinical research to identify the favorable and unfavorable innovations so that we may use the former and avoid the latter.

The statistics in Table 2 summarize the results.

TABLE 2   Analysis of Variance Estimates of Average and Standard Deviation of True Gains

	ESTIMATED AVERAGE GAIN	ESTIMATED STANDARD DEVIATION OF GAINS
Primary Therapies	1.5%	8%
Secondary Therapies	0.4%	21%

The average gain for the primary therapies is not far from zero, a result that agrees with our more qualitative analysis of Table 1. A zero average gain is consistent with some innovations having substantial improvements balanced by others having substantial losses or with other mixes such as many small gains and a few large losses. The size of the estimated standard deviation of effects of innovations lends added support to such interpretations. (A zero standard deviation would imply that all innovations give essentially the same amount of improvement.) And we know that some of these innovations do produce substantial improvements even when sample size is taken into account.

These figures also yield a rough guess about the proportion of comparisons having true differences favoring the innovation as great as, say, 10%. For the primary therapies, the probability that a new therapy has a positive gain of at least 10%, if the sample represents the future well, is about 0.13, or about 13 chances in 100.

For the secondary therapies, a gain of at least 10% (a 10% reduction in a specific complication) has a probability of 0.32.

The above procedure is rough and ready and leans hard upon an assumption of a normal distribution in its calculation, but the real distribution may not be normal. A new approach called "empirical Bayes" (Efron and Morris 1973) offers an alternative.

If each comparison were based on an infinitely large experiment, we would know the true gain exactly for that comparison. Then to estimate the proportion of gains of more than 10% we would count the number of comparisons with gains larger than 10% and divide by the total number of comparisons. And so if we had 25 comparisons and 5 had gains greater than 10%, we would estimate the probability of a gain of more than 10% as 5/25 or 0.20. This approach does not lean on any assumption about the shape of the distribution of true gains. But we can't use it because we do not have infinitely large experiments.

The new method takes note of the uncertainty associated with each observed gain, primarily using the sample sizes. Instead of regarding an observed gain as greater than 10%, or not greater, it estimates the probability that the true gain is greater than 10%. And so each comparison yields a probability of being greater than 10%, and we average these probabilities from all the comparisons to get our estimate of the overall probability of a gain of more than 10%.

If the observed gain is very large, say 30%, then its probability is nearly 1 (0.99, for example, or 99 chances out of 100) of having a true gain of more than 10% because the variability of the experimental observation is very much less than the 20% difference between 10% and 30%. This 0.99 corresponds to the 1 we would have counted toward the numerator (our 5 of the 5/25) had we known the true gain exactly. If the observed gain is negative, the probability that the true value exceeds 10% will be small, perhaps 0.01. This 0.01 is like the 0 we would have counted for this comparison had we known it to be exactly the true gain. When the observed gain is exactly 10%, the probability is 0.5 that the true gain is larger than 10% and 0.5 that it is smaller.

The same technique applies to finding the chance of gains greater than 5% or 0% or −7%, and so on. The resulting set of probabilities are conveniently graphed and thereby summarized by a cumulative distribution as shown in Figure 3.

Figure 5 shows the estimated cumulative distributions of the true gains in percentages for the primary and for the secondary therapies. By picking a gain in percentage, z, and reading the corresponding vertical axis on the appropriate curve, one can estimate the probability of a new therapy producing a gain as large as or larger than the chosen value of z.

For examples we have:

(a) For primary therapies the chances (i) of a 10% gain or more in survival are about 4 in 100 (we regard this as a better estimate than that given earlier [13 in 100] because we prefer the method rather than because we prefer the answer), (ii) of a 0% gain or more are about 48 in 100, (iii) of a loss of no more than 10% are about 98 in 100 which means that the chances of a loss in excess of 10% are about 2 in 100.

(b) For secondary therapies, the chances (i) of a gain of 10% or more in a specially chosen complication are estimated as 38 in 100 which is close to the earlier 32 in 100, (ii) of a 0% gain or more 57 in 100, (iii) of a loss of no more than 10% as 72 in 100, which means that a loss of 10% or more has chances of about 28 in 100.

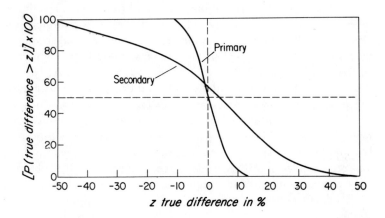

FIGURE 5

The Probability of a New Treatment Producing a Gain as Large as or Larger Than a Chosen Value, z

To find the probability of a difference in percentages greater than a given number z, say z = 10%, erect a perpendicular from 10% on the horizontal axis to the appropriate curve, and read its ordinate off the vertical axis, about 0.04 for the primary and about 0.38 for the secondary.

Is there some reason that secondary therapies are more likely to succeed than primary therapies? Is there something special about a treatment aimed at the disease process itself? We think the difference arises in large measure because in our quantitative analysis we chose to analyze primary therapies in which survival was an appropriate measure of outcome, while for secondary therapies the measure was avoidance of a specific complication. In a way the incidence of a specified complication is a much more discrete measure. One can envision a treatment having a large effect on a specific complication, whereas the difference between life and death may be the sum of the effects of a variety of factors—the primary treatment, the primary disease process, secondary treatments, and a variety of other disease processes and factors like old age and inter-current disease. Over the last generation the expected length of life has increased only slightly, but great changes have occurred in the variety and extent of postoperative complications as a result of changes in therapy such as the introduction of antibiotics, and of newer anesthetic agents, and techniques.

The sample of published papers is objectively chosen, and we think rather a good one for reflecting the sorts of differences analyzed here. What is less clear is how good a sample it is of therapeutic surgical research on patients generally during this period. First it is likely, and those we have talked with agree, that published papers are reports on better work on the average than that in unpublished research. Second, research that turns out well, our discussants agree, is more likely to be published. This reasoning suggests that the mass of unpublished research, insofar as it might produce measures comparable to those described in this paper, would have a lower average performance for innovations compared with standards than those in our sample. We suppose then that the innovations assessed by randomized clinical trials and reported in the surgical literature, and here, are biased upwards—that is, they present a more promising picture for innovation than if all innovations were subjected to randomized clinical trials. No doubt some innovations are so unsatisfactory that they are quickly abandoned, along with whatever trials were initiated on them. These conjectures suggest that if one were to consider adjusting the distributions shown in Figure 3 to report on all surgical innovations versus standards, the mean of the distribution would be lower and the standard deviation would probably be larger to allow for more frequent large negative differences. We have no grounds but speculation for the amount of such changes.

In a recent review of randomized trials used in evaluating social programs (Gilbert, Light, and Mosteller, 1976), the authors concluded that many new programs do not work and the effects of those that do are usually small. In contrast to these findings in the area of social innovations, this review provides strong evidence for a more optimistic view of the rate of progress in surgery and anesthesia. Almost half of the innovations reported in this series of controlled trials were at least as good as the standard, and a fair number were substantially better. Thus the analyses suggest that four out of ten innovations in secondary therapy produce a reduction in complication rates of 10% or more while two or three out of ten innovations in primary therapy produce a 5% or greater increase in survival. These estimates are for the distribution of the underlying true effects of the innovations. In a sense these results describe the clinical judgment that chooses those innovations as promising enough to test. If innovations were successful in a high proportion of trials, it would suggest that new therapies were being delayed until we were absolutely sure of their success, while if almost none were successful it would suggest a scarcity of new ideas in the field. Thus these distributions also describe research productivity and its effects on the development of better clinical care.

Another view is that this research process tries to reject all the innovations that produce losses and to keep the ones with gains. If this were done, then the median gain (the middle gain) retained for the primary therapies would be about 4%, and that for the secondary therapies would be about 15%. Of course, this would be an idealized state, for we cannot hope to weed out *all* the losses and detect *all* the gains. But it gives an estimated upper limit to what could be accomplished.

We further emphasize that to say that a proportion of innovations are substantial improvements does not serve to identify which they are.

Our findings give us an idea of the sorts of gains that can be made from selecting the better of pairs of therapies that are tested by randomized trials (we do not discuss the others here). The left sides of the curves warn us also that innovations may lose rather than gain, and so evaluation is needed. For example, in secondary therapies losses of as much as 20% could occur about one-fifth of the time. These curves emphasize the size and frequency of the losses as well as the gains. Thus as physicians well know, one cannot assume in advance that a new treatment is an improvement over an old, even when it looks promising enough to warrant a clinical trial. Our distributions show that some innovations provide important gains for the clinical care of patients, such as reducing a death rate by 5%.

To give an idea of the risks represented by a five percent change in death rate, we note that among all the people who died in recent years, 5% were in the ten year age range 40–49. Thus we can think of this rate as corresponding to the natural losses over a ten year period at middle age. Another way to think of 5% is that it is about four times the average surgical death rate from all operations over the country as a whole. Thus its importance is not small.

Reducing a death rate from 35% to 30% may be an important improvement in patient care, but this does not mean that it will be easily identified in the everyday setting of clinical practice. Indeed, statistical theory shows that a well-run randomized controlled trial would need 1,105 patients in each group to be 80% confident of detecting such a difference. Without a large formal trial, the uncontrolled effects of patient selection, of concurrent treatments, and of other factors make the detection of such differences even more difficult.

Since relatively small, even though important, numerical gains or losses are to be expected from most innovations, clinical trials must regularly be designed to detect these small differences accurately and reliably. Our sampled papers, taken as a group, provide an optimistic picture of progress in surgery and anesthesia. This progress depends on a judicious combination of continued development of new therapeutic ideas and their evaluation in good-sized unbiased clinical trials.

PROBLEMS

1.   What are the three basic types of studies reported in the sampled papers reviewed by the authors?

2.   Describe the scale used in the evaluation of the innovations.

3.   What is meant by primary and secondary therapies?

4.   Why is it not appropriate to consider a complete enumeration of papers during a certain period of time (say, 1964–1972) as a census rather than as a sample?

5.   Using Figure 3, calculate the estimated probability of an innovation being an improvement over the standard. (Hint: In what fraction of the 24 observed differences was I an improvement over S?)

6.   Find the estimated probability of an innovation being an improvement over the standard using Figure 4.

7.   Does a 0% average gain imply that all the innovations had exactly the same effect as the standards? Why, or why not?

8.   Why do the authors prefer the empirical Bayes method to the normal distribution method?

9.   Refer to Figure 5. In the primary therapies and in the secondary therapies what are the chances of
   a.   a gain of 30% or more?
   b.   a loss of no more than 20%?
   c.   a gain of more than 0%? Compare with the result for Problems 5 and 6.

10.   Why do the authors suppose that the innovations assessed by randomized clinical trials and reported in the surgical literature are "biased upwards"? What is meant by "biased upwards"?

REFERENCES

J. P. Gilbert, R. J. Light, and F. Mosteller, 1976. "Assessing Social Innovations: An Empirical Base for Policy." C. A. Bennett and A. R. Lumsdaine, eds., *Evaluation and Experiment: Some Critical Issues in Assessing Social Programs*. New York: Academic Press.

B. Efron and C. Morris, 1973. "Stein's Estimation Rule and its Competitors: An Empirical Bayes Approach." *Journal of the American Statistical Association*, 68: 117–130.

With permission of the Oxford University Press, this chapter is based on the longer article: J. P. Gilbert, B. McPeek, and F. Mosteller, "Progress in Surgery and Anesthesia: Costs, Risks, and Benefits of Innovative Therapy." J. P. Bunker, B. A. Barnes, and F. Mosteller, eds., *Costs, Risks, and Benefits of Surgery*, Oxford University Press, 1977.

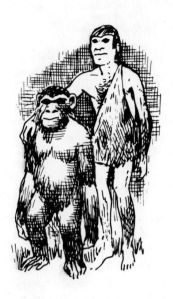

THE IMPORTANCE OF BEING HUMAN

W. W. Howells   *Harvard University*

IN THE summer of 1965, my paleontological colleague, Bryan Patterson, was in charge of a Harvard expedition working near the shore of Lake Rudolf in northern Kenya. At a locality called Kanapoi, searching in deposits believed to be of the early Pleistocene (the last geological epoch before the present), he picked up an important fossil. The broken lower end of a left humerus (the upper arm), it was easily recognized as *hominoid;* that is to say, it came from a creature of the group formed by man and his closest living relatives, the apes, but not from a monkey.

What was the special importance of the fossil? From shape and size it could be seen at once not to belong to a gorilla, an orangutan, or a gibbon (and the last two have never been present in Africa anyhow). It was extraordinarily similar to the same piece in modern man, in fact, it was indistinguishable. But the date of the deposit was certainly before the existence of anything like modern man, and after the field season was over, volcanic basalt from a bed lying above the deposit gave an age estimate, by radioisotope dating, of about 2½ million years. The oldest human stage that had been established so far was that of the erect-walking but small-brained and large-jawed australopithecines found by Leakey at Olduvai Gorge, which had been dated at about 1¾ million years. If this small piece of arm bone were "human," or *hominid,* in the sense of belonging to such a creature, it would extend the continuous record of human evolution backward three-quarters of a million years at a single bound.

But there was one problem. This piece of elbow joint in man can easily be told from that in orang, gorilla, and gibbon, but not from that in the chimpanzee. Although the rest of a chimpanzee's bone is shorter and stouter, this region is so similar in the two that many, if not most, specimens defy classification as one or the other on examination. In spite of different uses of the arm, this particular part shows such slight, subtle, and inconstant distinctions in size and shape as to baffle ordinary methods of study even by experts. The problem, therefore, was this: either the bone was that of the earliest australopithecine yet found in our direct ancestral history or it was simply that of an ancestral chimpanzee, in which case we could breathe normally. What about testing something old with something new? Could an electronic computer tell us anything useful?

A computer, of course, does not really "tell" anything. It merely makes possible answers to mathematical questions that we would not live long enough to answer if we tried to work them out with simple calculating machines. With its enormous capacities and speed, a computer transfers the effort from getting the right answer to getting the right question. Biological material— bones or skulls are good examples—lends itself to particular kinds of questions. Because the genes they inherit are capable of a virtually infinite number of different combinations, no two individuals of a population or species are exactly alike (with the spectacular exception of identical twins). So, quite apart from different habits of use, diet, or other accidents of growth, human elbow joints vary normally in size and details of shape, though they vary within a limit of form that is basic to the actions of human elbow joints.

Quite different species of animals, of course, have quite different forms in various body parts. Any beginner can distinguish between a cheek tooth of a mammalian carnivore, with its narrow, knifelike shearing crown, and that of a herbivore, which has a broad surface for grinding vegetable matter. These are marked evolutionary divergences. Within herbivores the differences are smaller, and within groups of herbivores such as pigs (for example, domestic pigs, wild boars, warthogs, etc.) or elephants, species distinctions are matters for experts, who can obtain a wealth of information from fossils as to the history of pigs and elephants or as to the exact species of animals present at a given time in the past at a fossil locality such as Kanapoi. Finally, for particular parts, such as the elbow joint in chimpanzee and man, the species distinctions may be so slight as to be eclipsed by the variation *within* each species, already described. That is the situation we are faced with here.

This is not just a matter of impression: it may be viewed quantitatively. Some time ago, Professor William L. Straus of Johns Hopkins University, a man with much experience in such studies, tried to deal with the same problem, when the same piece of the humerus of a species of australopithecine was found at the site of Kromdraai, near Pretoria, South Africa. In this case, it was plain that the bone belonged to *Paranthropus,* the species in question, because other skeletal and cranial parts of the same species had been found at the site, and the bone could hardly be assigned to anything else. Here the problem was whether the bone was more manlike or more apelike, since the hominid ("human") position of the australopithecines at that time was less clear. Professor Straus made a number of typical measurements of human and chimpanzee bones in an attempt to find differences between them. He found statistically significant differences[1] in the averages of certain of the measurements, but the absolute differences were slight, and the overlap in each measurement between man and chimp was so great that the *Paranthropus* fragment could not be allocated to either. In no case did its measurements lie outside the range of either man or chimpanzee, though the figures were more often closer to the mean, or average, figures for the latter.

This was no solution and led to no decision as to the relationships of *Paranthropus,* insofar as the arm could shed light on them. In such a case, we need a method that is not limited to comparisons of single measurements, but that somehow takes account of the whole shape of the bone, or part, as the eye tries to do, and also has some way of emphasizing the really telling differences in shape between two species, if they exist. Now here is an important point: in the end, any such problem comes down to a mathematical question because the eye itself (though very seldom consciously) attempts to assess the *average* differences in proportions and complex aspects of shape, to rate the varying importance of these, and finally, to judge the probability that a given total shape, in a single case, falls nearer to the essential basic form within the variation of one population than to that of another. These are questions of quantity and probability, whether measured or not, and are thus statistical in nature. After all, educated opinion is always the weighing of probabilities. And here is another important point: biologists and anthropologists—and members of many other sciences—are not often strong in mathematics of a higher order, though they may see only too acutely the limits of their own ways of solving problems. At the same time, mathematicians, although they have hearts of gold, are not usually sufficiently conversant

---

[1] The reader may recall that, when a statistician can detect a difference likely to be a real effect and not one stemming from chance variation, he calls it "statistically significant." By saying "statistically" he warns that the absolute size of the difference may be small and seemingly unimportant because it depends on the objects being studied.

with the niceties of biological problems to understand just what the biologist is trying to gain by using a mathematical analysis. When the two really get together, however, the rewards in the way of new solutions may be great. And I must say that mathematical training among biologists who see better what such training can offer has increased notably in recent years.

Fortunately, the particular problem of the Kanapoi fossil is not exceedingly complex, and the solution was provided some years ago by the great English statistician and geneticist R. A. Fisher in the form of the *discriminant function*. The discriminant function eliminates the futile business of looking at measurements one at a time, of finding that the overlap prevents discrimination of two sets of specimens such as human and chimp elbow joints even though they are known to be from quite different animals, and of being unable to place something such as the *Paranthropus* specimen logically nearer one group than the other. It has a set of weights with which to multiply a number of different measurements of a specimen, the sum of the products being a single *discriminant score* that makes the best attainable use of all the information in the several measurements. Given two groups, such as men and chimpanzees, the computation develops the optimum set of weights possible from the measurements used: the effect is to sift out important differences—often quite invisible to the eye or in average figures—so as to emphasize precisely the aspects of shape and size that will best discriminate between the two groups. That is to say, compared to just that variation *within* a set of human elbow joints, or chimpanzee elbow joints, the distinctions *between* the sets are searched out mathematically so that the discriminant scores of the two groups are segregated one from the other to the maximum degree possible, limited only by the information contained in the measurements. Thus the overlap, acting as a mask to hide any real group differences, is reduced or removed.

The basic idea of the discriminant function may be appreciated graphically in the case of *two* measurements, represented by the two axes of Figure 1. (The measurements might be heights and girths of two different groups of men.) The oval areas correspond to groups of individuals from two populations A and B. If we just look at measurement 1 by dropping projections on the horizontal axis, we find considerable overlap between the two populations. The same holds for measurement 2. On the other hand, the slanted line perfectly separates the two populations. This is not the place for mathematical detail, but to write the previous sentence is to say that looking at something like

(Measurement 1) + 2 × (Measurement 2)

gives us a new score, the discriminant score, which permits much better separation of the populations than either of measurements 1 or 2 alone. If there are more than two measurements, as in the present case, there are great potential gains in combining measurements.

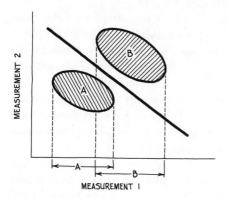

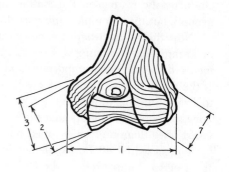

FIGURE 1

Two measurements together separate groups better than either separately

FIGURE 2

Kanapoi humeral fragment and measurements taken

Professor Patterson and I felt fairly strongly that the Kanapoi fragment was hominid—on the human, not the ape side, of the hominoid group as a whole. But we wanted to demonstrate this statistically, not merely to voice an opinion to which opposing opinions could be raised by others. As strategy, we examined human and chimpanzee humeri to see what measurements would most likely reflect such differences as we thought appeared, whether frequently or not. Figure 2 shows the fragment itself and some of the measurements. To begin with, we took the total breadth across the whole lower end, as a matter of general size (measurement 1). Second, the more projecting inner, or medial, epicondyle (at the left in the figure) has a snub-nosed, or slightly turned-up, aspect in some chimpanzees, and we hoped to register this effect by measuring from the lowest point on the trochlear ridge both to the "beak" of the epicondyle and to the nearest point on the shoulder just above it (measurements 2 and 3). The idea was that a slightly greater difference between these two would reflect a deeper curve and more upturned epicondyle. We also measured the backward protrusion of the central, or trochlear, ridge of the joint, the length and breadth of the oval inner face of the medial epicondyle (none of these is shown in Figure 2), and an oblique height of the opposite, or lateral, epicondyle. We thought these measurements showed some tendency to vary one way in man, the other in chimpanzees, though not being the rule in either (if there *were* regular distinctions, obviously the problem of discrimination would be much less). We were not certain of the functional meaning of the possible differences, but they logically could be related mostly to muscle attachments connected with simpler and more powerful use of the flexor and extensor muscles of the hand in the chimp, in hanging by the arms or supporting the body in ground-walking by the characteristic resting on the middle knuckles, all as contrasted with the more general, but more complex and varied, use of the hands in man.

Now this is just where the cooperation comes in. It is the paleontologist's or anthropologist's business, from his background knowledge, to find measurements that will carry important and real information as to differences. It is the statistician's business to say how the measurements can be put together to bring out the differences for evaluation. Here, cooperation had already gone so far in recent years that the biologists knew in advance what statisticians could offer them and we planned our work accordingly.

We measured 40 human bones in the Peabody Museum at Harvard and those of 40 chimpanzees in the Harvard Museum of Comparative Zoology and the American Museum of Natural History in New York. As in Straus's measurements, the overlap of man and chimp was great, but the mean differences, resulting from the special selection of measurements, were in most cases better defined. The means for the two groups and the figures for both the Kanapoi and Kromdraai fragments (the latter taken on two casts) are given to $\frac{1}{10}$ mm in Table 1.

The chimpanzee specimens, as a sample, may be accidentally a little large on the average. The *Paranthropus* fragment is obviously small in all dimensions and so appears "human" when we glance at this list; however, this does not necessarily mean that the shape relations conform to those of man. The correspondences of the Kanapoi measurements to the human means (of this particular sample) are very close throughout—closer than we might expect any random human bone to be in all its measurements.

To assure ourselves of this apparent closeness, we computed a discriminant function from the human and chimp figures. For only seven measurements and such small samples, the calculations could be done by hand, though at the cost of no little labor. In technical language, matrices have to be formed of the sums of all the cross multiplications of all the measurements of all the individuals both within each group and of the total lot; other

TABLE 1. Measurements

MEASUREMENT	CHIMP MEAN	HUMAN MEAN	KANA- POI	PARANTH- ROPUS	SCALED VECTOR
1. Bi-epicondylar width	64.1	58.0	60.2	53.6	− .09
2. Trochlea-med. epi. dist.	44.8	40.7	41.7	33.6	+ .40
3. Trochlea-supracond. dist.	41.3	38.8	39.4	32.1	− .62
4. Posterior trochlear edge	26.4	22.1	22.2	19.9	+ .11
5. Med. epi. length	24.7	20.3	20.8	15.5	+ .19
6. Med. epi. breadth	12.8	12.6	13.9	10.4	− .32
7. Lat. epi. height	31.5	26.7	27.6	24.9	+ .56

steps require the inversion of one matrix and the determination of the latent roots of another. Inversion by hand of a matrix of even the modest size of 7×7 is a tedious business and one open to error. This all leads to finding the discriminant function, which takes the seven measurements from a specimen, multiplies each measurement by a weight specific to that measurement, and then adds these products to give the discriminant score. This is a great deal of arithmetic and we can only say that to have a computer handle such a job from punched cards in a matter of minutes is very welcome. Waiting for paint to dry or for a film to be developed now seems long and drawn out by comparison, and such easy computation has obviously greatly encouraged undertakings such as the one described here.

The last column in Table 1 gives, not the actual weights in the discriminant function as used, but rather a rescaled form of the weights with their relative importance in proper perspective (because, for example, a small measurement, such as thumb length, might require a much larger weight in the function than a large measure, such as stature, to make it effective). These figures show how a number of measurements combine to form a single pattern of greatest difference between the two groups. As might have been expected, the two measurements to register the snub-nosed effect of the medial epicondyle, or its opposite, are useful, as shown by the large size of the scaled vector values. The plus value of measurement 2 and the minus value of measurement 3 combine to make the total discriminant score higher when the epicondyle is most turned up; that is, when measurement 2 is high relative to measurement 3 (see Figure 1), the function creates a greater positive value to add and a smaller minus value to subtract in the total score, and when the opposite is true, with the shoulder of the condyle more sloping, there is on balance a greater minus value in the total score. The lateral epicondyle (measurement 7) also adds a greater plus value when it is high, while the breadth of the medial epicondyle (measurement 6) adds to a plus value (or rather subtracts *least* from a total value) when it is relatively narrow.

Table 1 shows that the above are indeed characteristic human-chimp differences in the averages (though small ones), all of which tend to produce higher score values for the chimpanzee. We note that there is almost no *absolute* difference in measurement 6, the breadth of the medial epicondyle, certainly not a significant one, and yet this measurement is important in discrimination because it is *relatively* narrow in chimpanzees, whose other measurements (in these samples) are larger, on the average, than the human measurements.

We notice also that because the discriminant score is affected by all measurements, it takes account of variation in form toward or away from a basic pattern: if a chimpanzee bone lacks any snubbing of the medial epicondyle, it may exhibit another combination of narrow epicondylar face or high lateral epicondyle, and so it may score in a chimpanzee direction anyhow.

When the discriminant scores were calculated, they produced a far greater separation of human and chimpanzee bones than did any of the measurements singly. Here are the mean score values, and the limits of the individuals in each group:

	Mean	Range
Chimpanzee	99.77	67–130
Man	61.42	40–84

All but two of the chimpanzee values fall between 80 and 120, and all but one of the human values fall between 50 and 75, which are nonoverlapping intervals. So the separation was very good: of 80 specimens, only three overlapped, falling closer to the wrong mean figure than to their own. Unquestionably, this is a successful procedure to distinguish human and chimpanzee humeri by measurement, with a much greater probability of correct assignment than is possible by eye.

Now for the scores of the Kanapoi and *Paranthropus* fragments. These were 59.4 and 63.9, respectively, very close to the human average (almost too good to be true, being closer than most of the known human individuals) and, of course, outside the range of the 40 chimpanzee values entirely. Using statistical theory we compute that, had either bone actually belonged to a chimpanzee, it would have a discriminant score as small as those above (or smaller) with a probability of only about 1 in 500. With so small a probability, we conclude that the two bones did not come from chimpanzees, but from hominids, and that is the answer to the question we framed.

Of course, we must be careful. The real question (because of the material we used) was this: how do the fragments classify themselves when they are asked to choose between *modern* human and *modern* chimpanzee arm bones? These were the only alternatives which we offered to fossil creatures which existed when there were no modern men, and when ancestral chimpanzees might also have differed significantly from those of today. Nevertheless, we have good grounds for inferring from their shape that the arm bones were used, on the whole, like those of men and, at least, not like those of the African apes, terrestrial though they are to a great extent. This takes care of the Kanapoi individual and, as a bonus, says the same thing for the hitherto baffling fragment from Kromdraai.

To review: unable to establish from visual inspection that the Kanapoi fossil did not belong to an animal like a chimpanzee, we turned to measurement and a statistical procedure that could be applied with the help of a computer. (As biologists, we knew from experience how to state the problem and extract a great deal of information, but how to order, analyze, and judge it we learned from statisticians.) Though moderately complex, the discriminant function is well suited to the biological realities of individual variation and group differences in shape and gives an answer that states a numerical probability from the known evidence. So, by the middle of 1966, Professor Patterson and I had concluded that we could rule out the possibility that he had found the bone of an ape and that from what we know about East Africa, the only other possible possessor of the fossil was an early hominid, that is, an australopithecine.

Happy though this made us, the original question since has become partly academic. Patterson went back to the Lake Rudolf region and other teams have been at work in fossil-bearing areas to the north. It is now clear to Patterson (from such evidence as fossil pigs and elephants and more radio-isotope dates) that the Kanapoi formation is over 4 million years old, not 2½ million. Numerous australopithecine fossils—skulls, jaws, teeth, leg bones— have been found in different places with ages of 1 to 4 million years; and at a locality known as Lothagam Hill, near Lake Rudolf, Patterson found a piece of a lower jaw that is clearly hominid, that is, another early australopithecine, and that is over 5 million years old. So it has to be accepted that the Kanapoi bone is that of an australopithecine, agreeing with the result obtained from the disciminant function.

If the original question now has less meaning, our analysis also implies something about the actual form of the bone: it was used in human fashion. This is equally important, if not more so. Several anthropologists and graduate students have recently been using similar, but more complex, analyses to study shape and function of other bones and fragments of our early ancestors, the australopithecines.

PROBLEMS

1. In the hypothetical example of Figure 1, project the values of measurement 2 for groups A and B onto the vertical axis and indicate the interval where the two populations overlap on measurement 2. Using Figure 1 explain why one needs to look at both measurements (or a function of these measurements) to be able to classify an individual as being in A or B.

2. Suppose instead of the two populations in Figure 1 we have the populations in Figure 3 below. It is then very easy to discriminate between the two populations. How would you do it?

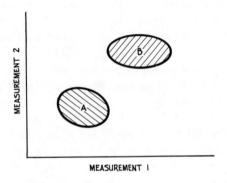

MEASUREMENT 1

Figure 3

Using this example and the one in Figure 1 explain when discriminant functions are needed.

3. In Table 1 note that there is almost no difference in measurement 6 for humans and chimpanzees, yet it was one of the measurements to help discriminate between the two populations. Explain how measurement 6 might help in discriminating between the two populations.

4. Give a detailed example of your own in which a discriminant function analysis might be appropriate.

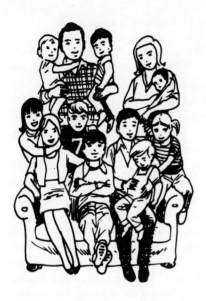

HOW CROWDED WILL WE BECOME?

Nathan Keyfitz   *University of California, Berkeley*

ALL STATISTICAL facts concern the past. The Census of April 1970 counted
205 million of us, but we did not know this until November, despite the
census emphasis on speed, pursued with ingenuity and with much new electronic equipment. Stock-market prices and volumes are hours old before
they appear in the evening paper. Statistics of plans or intentions are only
an apparent exception. No one can ever gather data directly on the future.

Yet the actions that statistics serve to guide can occur only in the future.
The local telephone company wants to know how much this town will grow
in population over the next few decades. Its interest is not abstract curiosity,
but contemplated construction of new lines out toward a certain suburb. The
investment might occur in the next two or three years, and the service given
by the investment along with the income derived from it would be spread
over 30 years. If the town does not grow as much as expected, the construction would be wasteful. If the growth is in the direction of a different suburb,
then lines will be idle on one side of the town and too often busy on the other

side.   School authorities, the bus company, a textile manufacturer, all similarly need statistics on the future for the conduct of their business, and these are nowhere to be collected until the future has become past and it is too late.

With producers of population statistics all working on the near side of *now* and users all concerned with the far side, it is lucky that even in times of rapid change, some continuities are to be found between past and future. Population projection rests on these continuities.

The continuities are not be found in simple totals.   We know that the number of people in the U.S. does not increase evenly from year to year, and still less does the population of one town or one age group increase evenly.   The age classes especially have fluctuated erratically in recent decades.   Today the U.S. includes an exceptionally large proportion of young people 10 to 25 years of age, the result of the baby boom of the forties and fifties.   They have crowded the high schools and colleges, and they are seeking jobs and entry into graduate schools across the country.   But during the sixties, births fell sharply, and the number of pupils entering elementary schools leveled off.

Yet we can say something about the future.   At the end of the seventies, schools and the labor market will be reached by the wave of what may be called the nonbirths of the sixties.   But, though kindergartens and public schools will slow their expansion in the seventies, they may have to accelerate it again in the eighties to accommodate a new generation—children of the children born in the postwar baby boom.   How such things can be projected with some confidence is our subject.

The approach, or model, that we shall build for projection serves other purposes than prediction.   It is especially valuable for judging the effects on population growth of a possible change or a proposed policy.

PROJECTION WITH CONSTANT BIRTH AND DEATH RATES

The trick in projection is to seek elements that remain nearly constant through time.   The increase in total population from year to year plainly does not qualify, but certain *rates* do remain more or less the same, and on these we rest our analysis of the future.   For example, the proportion of people aged 30 who die each year is likely to remain much the same in 1960, 1970, and 1980.   These death rates are constant enough that some fairly reliable predictions can be hung on them, and we proceed to the exploitation of this constancy.

Our projection of population into the future includes three parts:

(1) The statistical data of a baseline census from which work starts
(2) Effect of death
(3) Effect of birth

Demographers ordinarily recognize five-year age groups, to the end of life, for men and women separately, and they have a computer do the arithmetic. To show the procedure without being swamped in numbers, we consider here girls and women only, and these just up to age 45. Moreover, we need only consider three age groups, each of 15 years' width. For purposes of this illustration, three numbers describe the population at any one time.

We can make a fairly complete analysis for these three groups, and show the whole worksheet. The census of April 1, 1960, counted 27.4 million girls under 15 in the U.S. It showed only 17.7 million between 15 and 29 years. An intermediate number, 18.4 million, were between 30 and 44. (This article follows the census in always counting people at their age last birthday.) Those under 15, born between 1945 and 1960, constitute the baby boom; the next older group, born between 1930 and 1945, are survivors of the meager crop of depression babies; the oldest, aged 30 to 44, were born between 1915 and 1930, when birth rates in the U.S. were higher than in the thirties, but lower than in the fifties.

Now these three numbers can be written one below another in an array known as an age distribution; see Table 1.

So much for the counts made in 1960, our point of takeoff into the future. We now need to know how death and birth will act on this starting distribution. (Migration, which demographers usually take into account in making projections, is probably going to be relatively small and not likely to affect our conclusions seriously, so we shall ignore it.)

Let us start with death, but look at its positive side: the people who do not die, but survive into the next period. The question is, how many of the 27.4 million girls under 15 years of age counted in the 1960 census may be expected to survive to 1975? We have at hand a *life table,* as such collections of survival probabilities are called, that gives the proportion of girls under 15 who survive for 15 years as approximately 0.9924. This life table was calculated from deaths in the U.S. in 1965, and it would not be very different if calculated for any other recent year. Hence the expected number of survivors 15 years later of the 27.4 million counted in 1960 would be

TABLE 1. Age Distribution of American Girls and Women, 1960

AGE	MILLIONS OF GIRLS AND WOMEN
0–14	27.4
15–29	17.7
30–44	18.4

27.4 multiplied by 0.9924, or 27.2 million. These girls would be 15 to 29 years of age in 1975.

No such multiplication can give the *exact* numbers in 1975. Individuals survive or die at random, and even if 0.9924 were the probability for each separate girl 0–14 years of age, a few more or a few less than 27.4 × 0.9924 million could survive in the particular years 1960–75. If the U.S. were subject to serious epidemics, chance events each affecting large numbers of people, then the variation from year to year would be substantial. Because, in fact, death and survivorship act like events affecting each of us more or less independently, the multiplication is permissible, though even then the result could be made wrong by a war or epidemic on the one hand or a medical breakthrough on the other. We shall suppose that the chance of survival does not change very greatly over the period of the projection.

In the same way the proportion surviving 15 years among girls 15 to 29 in 1960 is estimated at 0.9826, and hence the projected number aged 30 to 44 in 1975 would be 17.7 × 0.9826 = 17.4 million. The projections to this point stand as shown in Table 2. Our next task is to fill the upper cell on the right, which requires an estimate of the number under 15 in 1975. (Remember that, to keep things manageable and simple, we are neglecting women 45 or more—of course, only for present simplicity, as the wives of some of us will remind us.)

All of the girls under 15 years of age in 1975 will have been born since 1960, and we need to estimate not how many girl births take place in the 15 years, but how many of these births survive to 1975. We know, also from the 1965 experience, that, on the average a woman 15 to 29 can expect 0.8498 surviving girl babies by the end of a 15-year period. We have counted girl babies only for this purpose because a female model is what we are constructing, and we have deducted deaths among the babies so as to come up with girls under 15 who will be alive in 1975. There were 17.7 million women aged 15 to 29 in 1960, and their contribution to the total girls under 15 in 1975 is expected to be 17.7 × 0.8498 = 15.0 million.

TABLE 2. Projected 1975 Population of American Girls and Women

AGE	MILLIONS OF GIRLS AND WOMEN	
	1960	1975
0–14	27.4	?
15–29	17.7	27.2
30–44	18.4	17.4

Children will be born also to the women 30 to 44 years of age; on the average, these women will have 0.1273 girl babies alive at the end of the 15-year period. The contribution that these make to the total girls under 15 in 1975 is expected to be $18.4 \times 0.1273 = 2.4$ million. (The actual calculation was made to more decimals than shown here.)

Finally, children will be born before 1975 to girls under 15 in 1960, a large proportion of whom will become of childbearing age during the 15 years. On the average (again at 1965 rates), they will have 0.4271 surviving girls. This average, like the others above, is taken over many different cases; it includes the girls too young to become mothers, those who will be old enough but not yet married, and those who will marry but not have children. The expected contribution here is $27.4 \times 0.4271 = 11.7$ million.

To find the total number of girl children under 15 surviving in 1975 we must add the numbers reached in the three preceding paragraphs: $11.7 + 15.0 + 2.4 = 29.1$ million in all. Figure 1 shows schematically what is happening. (Because so few children are born to women over 44, we can afford to ignore them. Our simple model will give almost the same rate of increase of the population as more elaborate models.)

By repeating exactly the same argument, except that we now start with the 1975 projected population, we obtain the age distribution in 1990; any

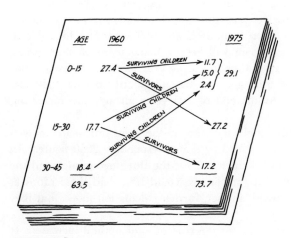

FIGURE 1

Calculation of 1975 population of girls and women under 45 years of age (figures are in millions)

TABLE 3. Millions of Girls and Women Under 45 Years of Age in the U.S. if Birth and Death Rates Remain at the 1965 Level

AGE	1960	1975	1990	2005	2020	2035	2050	2065
0–14	27.4	29.1	37.7	44.1	54.3	65.0	79.0	95.3
15–29	17.7	27.2	28.9	37.5	43.7	53.8	64.5	78.4
30–44	18.4	17.4	26.7	28.4	36.8	43.0	52.9	63.4
Total	63.5	73.7	93.3	110.0	134.8	161.8	196.4	237.1

number of additional 15-year cycles may be calculated similarly.   Table 3 shows the resulting numbers up to 2065.

WAVES OF MOTHERHOOD

The first age group, girls under 15, increases less than two million between 1960 and 1975, while the women 15 to 29 increase by almost 10 million.   The 15 to 29 group in 1975 are the babies born between 1945 and 1960, the postwar baby boom, and as these succeed the depression babies in any group we expect its number to rise rapidly.   Women 30 to 44 actually become fewer during this first 15-year period, even though the 0 to 44 population as a whole is growing.

Because most children are born to mothers 15 to 29 years of age, we can expect a new baby boom, an echo of the first one, at the time when the babies of the fifties themselves pass through childbearing age, and indeed the under-15s grow by 8.6 million from 1975 to 1990 according to Table 3.

In fact, the depression and boom will keep echoing to much later times, supposing, as we do throughout, that childbearing practices remain fixed.   But the table also shows that as time goes on the irregularity of the 1960 age distribution steadily lessens.   At the end of 105 years all ages are increasing at very nearly the same rate.

That the several ages ultimately increase at the same rate can be seen by dividing each 2065 figure in Table 3 by the corresponding 2050 figure.   In Table 4, this ratio is shown to be about 1.2 for the three age groups and the total.   By carrying the projection further, we could have had these ratios as close to one another as we wanted; in fact, further calculation shows that they all would converge to 1.2093.

This ratio may be called intrinsic, or the true ratio of natural increase.   It can be shown to depend not at all on the 1960 age distribution with which the process started, but only on the rates of birth and death, and it is the most informative single summary measure of that set of rates.   It tells us that any population that is subject to our particular birth and death rates

TABLE 4. Increase of Age Groups of Girls and Women in the U.S. from 2050 to 2065

AGE	2050 (MILLIONS)	2065 (MILLIONS)	RATIO, 2065 TO 2050
0–14	79.0	95.3	1.206
15–19	64.5	78.4	1.216
30–44	52.9	63.4	1.198
Total	196.4	237.1	1.207

over a period of time will sooner or later settle down to an increase in the ratio 1.2093, which is to say by about 21% per 15-year period. Under the operation of the projection, applying the assumptions we have made, *a stable age distribution* is sooner or later attained in which all the irregularities of 1960 due to boom and depression have been forgotten. Age distributions tend to forget their past when persistently pushed forward by the method developed above.

Let us find numerically the component of population growth that increases in the same ratio in every cycle, a mode of increase spoken of as *geometric*. If we divide each of the numbers shown under the year 2065 in Table 3 by 1.2093, we get back to an estimate for 2050; if we then divide again by 1.2093 we get back to 2035, and so on. To get back to 1960 we would divide by the seventh power of 1.2093, written $(1.2093)^7$ and equal to 3.78. Carrying out the division gives 95.3/3.78 or 25.2 million for age 0 to 14, and similar calculations for the other ages provide what we may call the stable equivalent for 1960; see Table 5.

Table 5 shows the set of numbers that, increasing in the constant ratio 1.2093, would sooner or later exactly join the track of our projection in each age group. If we multiply the stable equivalent by the fixed number 1.2093 to obtain the geometric track, and subtract this from the projection of Table

TABLE 5. Main Component of Female Population in the U.S., 1960

AGE	STABLE EQUIVALENT (MILLIONS)
0–14	25.2
15–29	20.7
30–44	16.8
Total	62.7

TABLE 6. Departures of Projected
Population in Table 3 from Geometric
Progression in Millions

AGE	1960	1975	1990	2005
0–14	2.2	−1.4	0.9	−0.6
15–29	−3.0	2.2	−1.4	0.9
30–44	1.6	−2.9	2.1	−1.4

3, we obtain Table 6. For example, for girls 0 to 14 in 1975, we have
$29.1 - 25.2 \times 1.2093 = -1.4$. Our analysis has separated the prospective
population change into two parts, one a smooth geometric increase, the other
a series of waves that are departures from the geometric.

These departures gradually diminish in amplitude. For 1960, we have
2.2 million as a measure of the temporary "excess" of the 1945–60 babies.
The −3.0 million are the deficiency of the depression babies, and 1.6 million,
again an excess, relate to the twenties. Note that by 1990, each of these
has an echo, of the same sign but on the whole of smaller amount.

The tendency of the waves to diminish in amplitude is related to women
having their children over a range of ages. If all children were born to
mothers of the same age, the waves would steadily *increase* in amplitude.
With such concentration any irregularity in the age distribution caused, for
example, by a war or depression would not only continue echoing through
all later generations, but become magnified. In the U.S. today, women
prefer to have their children around age 25, whereas our grandmothers spread
theirs from about 20 to 45. The new style, associated with the effective
use of birth control, could mean diminished stability.

In this analysis of the U.S. population we have gone from the facts
of the 1960 census, through various more or less realistic calculations concerning 1975 and even 1990, into a kind of fantasy as we proceed far into the
future. The early part of the projection can within limits be useful for practical purposes; the later part is so dependent on various *if's* that one would
be very foolish to count on it. The biggest doubt attaches to the birth rate.
It may seem that birth is as individual a matter as death, and therefore
births across the country ought to be independent of one another, yet in
fact high and low birth rates spread like epidemics across the country.

Why then do we bother with the fantasy of such far-out projections referring to the distant future? The answer is that they help us understand
the present. We ascertain the meaning of the present rates of birth and
death by calculating what they *would* lead to if they continued for a hundred
years or more. Let us see why this is even more important in study of the

birth and death rates of developing countries than of a developed one like the U.S.

GROWTH OF DEVELOPING COUNTRIES

The task is in some ways easier for developing countries because they do not have a history of changing birth rates. It is true that their death rates have been falling, and where this occurs for young children only, it is the equivalent of a rise in the birth rate: as far as the population mathematics is concerned, a fall in infant deaths has the same effect as a rise in births. In fact, however, deaths have been falling at nearly all ages, and births are relatively unchanged. The fact is that age distributions are already more or less in the condition we called stable, and which could be attained by the U.S. only in the course of several generations of fixed rates. Because of past uniformly high birth rates, developing countries tend to grow much faster than the U.S. Moreover, they show a simple geometric increase, with all ages rising uniformly. The sort of waves that we have been studying do not occur for them.

Let us concentrate then on the geometric component, and take Malaysia as an example. In the mid-sixties, Malaysia was growing in the intrinsic ratio defined above of 1.59 per 15 years. This corresponds to an annual rate of increase of the 15th root of 1.59 or 1.031, that is, about 3.1% per year, against about 1% for the U.S. To convince ourselves of this we could multiply 1.031 by itself 15 times, that is calculate $(1.031)^{15}$, and we would find the result to be just under 1.59.

We can see the long-term prospect more clearly by translating into doubling times. How long does it take a country that is increasing at the rate r % per year to double in population? The equation to be solved for the unknown time t is $[1 + (r/100)]^t = 2$. The solution is obtained by taking logarithms of both sides and comes out very near to $t = 70/r$, where r is expressed as percent increase. This rule applies to money lent out at interest, and financiers use it because they are very interested in doubling times. The same sort of rule works for the half-life of a piece of radium or other substance under radioactive decay.

As an example of a geometric projection of a population, suppose that Malaysia's rate of 3.1% per year were to go on for about $70/3.1 = 23$ years. This would carry it from the present 10 up to 20 million people. Suppose it went on for another 23 years; this would mean another doubling. At the end of 115 years at this rate, the population would have doubled five times, which means multiplying by 2^5 or 32; Malaysia would contain 320 million persons. By the end of 230 years, it would have doubled ten times and would contain 2^{10} times as many as now, or 1024 times ten million.

No one could mistake such calculations for predictions of what will happen. In a sense they are the opposite; we might call them counterpredictions, for they show that in much less than 100 years, the birth rate will go down or the death rate will go up or both. Most demographers are optimistic enough to believe that the adjustment will be through the birth rate.

Other countries are today growing faster than Malaysia. Mexico's present 50 million population is increasing at about 3.5% per year, which, by our rule, would give it a doubling time of $70/3.5 = 20$ years. At this rate, it would be 100 million by the year 1990, 200 million by the year 2010, and 400 million by the year 2030. This again is a counterprediction; shortage of food, excess of pollution, and many other reasons would prevent it from coming true. The usefulness of the calculation is in showing that births must be reduced; anyone who makes a *principle* of permanent opposition to birth control in effect favors an increase of the death rate sooner or later. The most that opponents of birth control can argue is that it should be delayed a few years.

In diluted form, the same is true of the U.S. Our calculation showed that the geometric component, neglecting waves, was an increase of 21% for 15 years, or about 1.2% per year, according to births and deaths of 1965. That means a doubling in 60 years, quadrupling in 120 years, and so on. Contract the U.S. time scale by about three, and the future growth of the U.S. is the same as that of Mexico. And even our having three years to Mexico's one is partly offset by the greater damage to the environment caused by our more advanced industry.

RELIABILITY OF PREDICTION

The techniques presented in this article and obvious extensions of them are much used for predicting the future. They are used not because they are perfect, but because nothing better is available. Whatever continuities exist in birth and death rates are exploited by the makers of projections. From about 1870 to 1935 in Western Europe and the U.S., the birth rate and the death rate were both falling; projections could be made by the method outlined here, except that instead of using fixed rates, the past downward trend in birth and death was projected into the future. Such projections were acceptably accurate as long as the downward trend continued.

But these same countries reached a turning point in the forties. People married younger, and births rose rapidly. Moreover, couples varied the timing of their children as well as varying the total number. The fact that in a modern society couples plan their children, both in number and in timing, can be used to strengthen the predictions. Samples of young couples are surveyed to find what their childbearing intentions are, just as we ask intentions on buying houses and automobiles. The official estimates of the U.S. Bureau of the Census take account of these intentions.

The Census Bureau's projections, which use a vastly elaborated form of the method of this article, can be compared with ours. Theirs are more detailed than ours above have been, and they are also cautious enough to make a variety of projections rather than betting on just one. They end up with four numbers for each age, sex, and future year. For example, for 1990, their four numbers for girls 0 to 14 years of age range from a low of 29.5 million to a high of 41.8 million. Our Table 3 shows 37.7 million.

How well would past application of our model have foretold the 1970 population of the U.S.? If we had worked forward from the 1920 census total of 106 million, using exactly the procedure of this article, but applying it in five-year age intervals to all ages and to both sexes, we would have found about 185 million for 1970. If we had allowed for immigration less emigration of 200,000 per year, this would have brought us to 195 million against the 205 million actually counted. Something a little lower would have been found starting from 1950; starting from 1960, we would have slightly overestimated the census figure. An error of about 5% in estimates made up to 50 years ago is not bad, considering that the Bureau of the Census estimates its own actual count to be subject to nearly 2% error.

We would have done much worse starting in 1940, however; the method of this essay, plus about 6 million immigrants, would have produced a total of only about 160 million. Put another way that sounds even worse: the increase from 1940 to 1970 was about 62 million, and of it, we would have estimated less than 30 million. This is not a good score. The baby boom of the fifties was a historic event about as hard to predict in advance as the war that sparked it.

MODELS PERMIT EXPERIMENTS

We have discussed the population projection as a way of making predictions, and also as a way of making counterpredictions—calculating what would happen if present rates continued as a way of showing that they cannot continue. This last suggests what may be the most important use of the model of this essay, originally developed and still often applied to making predictions. This use is experimentation. Not only does our model answer the question "What would happen if the birth and death rates of the present time continue into the future?" but it answers a great variety of other important questions. What would be the effect on total population numbers if intensive research on heart disease was undertaken, and it reduced deaths from that cause by 90%? This could conceivably result from a research effort comparable to present investigations of outer space. But the effort could equally be put into reduction of infant mortality. Our model could compare the effects of these alternatives, taking account of the fact that the person dying of heart disease is of such an age that he will soon die of something else; the child saved from some lethal ailment, on the average, will have a long life ahead of him. A given fall in infant mortality increases the population by much more than the same fall in heart disease.

An example of a question that has been frequently asked, and to which our model provides a clear answer, is: what would happen if, starting now, each member of the population averaged one descendant? This means that each fertile couple would need to have somewhat more than two children, to allow for those who do not marry, for those who marry but are infertile, and for deaths in childhood. An average of about 2.3 children per married couple would constitute bare replacement, that is to say, would keep the population stationary at modern death rates.

But the stationary *level* at which it would keep it would be above that of the starting point. Any population that has been subject to birth rates higher than bare replacement in the past has a large proportion of girls and women of childbearing age. These will produce increasing numbers of children for about 50 years after the date at which the birth rate falls. The projection model developed in this article tells how high the population would rise if we drop to bare replacement numbers of children.

Application of the model shows that the U.S. would rise to about 270 million persons if bare replacement were adopted today, and Mexico would rise from its present 50 million to over 80 million. Most underdeveloped countries, such as Mexico, would increase by about 65% from the point at which they drop to replacement, and they would do this over 50 or so years. No country ought to fear that immediate adoption of contraception would freeze total population where it stands; a kind of momentum operates simply because of the favorable age distribution that results from past high fertility.

Former President Sukarno of Indonesia was against birth control because he thought Indonesia should have 250 million people. The present government applied the model described in this essay and found it will probably exceed 250 million even if the brakes are put on immediately; consequently it has formally sponsored a program of birth control.

CONCLUSION

We started this essay by developing a model to forecast the future. The model works for forecasts over short periods and over longer periods in which either the trend is steady or in which ups and downs offset one another. For forecasting major turning points it is of little use, but so is any other model so far developed.

While the model is moderately, but only moderately, successful for the purpose for which it is designed, it has the power to analyse hypothetical futures whose consideration is urgent. If the marriage age in India is raised to 20, what effect will this have on the birth rate? If 20% of couples aged

30 accept sterilization, how far will this take a given country towards zero population growth? How much long-run effect does the emigration from Jamaica have on its population increase? What kind of population waves would follow a sudden drop in the birth rate of an underdeveloped country? It is in answering questions such as these, of which examples have been given in the course of this essay quite as much as in making predictions, that the projection model presented here finds its use.

PROBLEMS

1. What is a "life-table"?

2. What assumptions must one make to be able to predict, with some accuracy, the future population size using a life table?

3. In Table 2, why cannot one use the same method to calculate the three entries in the last column?

4. What is meant by "diminished stability" as a result of the new style of childbirth associated with the effective use of birth control?

5. Give some reasons why the method of prediction used in the article might give biased results.

6. What is the usefulness of the proposed model of population growth? Describe a few questions for which the model can provide answers.

7. Using the stable equivalent for 1960 females in the age group 0–14 given in Table 5, we can get the stable equivalent for the year 2065 of the same age group by multiplying 25.2 by $(1.2093)^7$.
    a. What power of 1.2093 should 25.2 be multiplied by to get the stable equivalent for the year 1990? Calculate this number.
    b. Is the stable equivalent obtained for 1990 in part a. equal to 37.7 (the number given in Table 3)? If not, how big is the difference? Compare with the difference 0.9 shown in Table 6.

8. Verify the numbers in the column for the year 2065 of Table 3 using the method given in the text in connection with Table 2.

9. Verify the solutions for the doubling time $t=70/r$ of the equation $(1+(r/100))^t=2$. If the growth rate of a country is 2%, what is the doubling time?

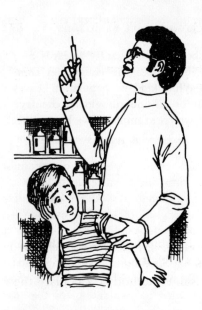

THE BIGGEST PUBLIC HEALTH EXPERIMENT EVER: The 1954 Field Trial of the Salk Poliomyelitis Vaccine

Paul Meier *University of Chicago*

THE LARGEST and most expensive medical experiment in history was carried out in 1954. Well over a million young children participated, and the immediate direct costs were over 5 million dollars. The experiment was carried out to assess the effectiveness, if any, of the Salk vaccine as a protection against paralysis or death from poliomyelitis. The study was elaborate in many respects, most prominently in the use of placebo controls (children who were inoculated with simple salt solution) assigned at random (that is, by a carefully applied chance process that gave each volunteer an equal probability of getting vaccine or salt solution) and subjected to a double-blind evaluation (that is, an arrangement under which neither the children nor the physicians who evaluated their subsequent state of health knew who had been given vaccine and who got the salt solution).

Why was such elaboration necessary? Did it really result in more or better knowledge than could have been obtained from much simpler studies? These are the questions on which this discussion is focused.

BACKGROUND

Polio was never a common disease, but it certainly was one of the most frightening and, in many ways, one of the most inexplicable in its behavior. It struck hardest at young children, and, although it was responsible for only about 6% of the deaths in the age group 5 to 9 in the early fifties, it left many helpless cripples, including some who could survive only in a respirator. It appeared in epidemic waves, leading to summer seasons in which some communities felt compelled to close swimming pools and restrict public gatherings as cases increased markedly from week to week; other communities, escaping an epidemic one year, waited in trepidation for the year in which their turn would come. Rightly or not, this combination of selective attack upon the most helpless age group and the inexplicable vagaries of its epidemic behavior, led to far greater concern about polio as a cause of death than other causes, such as auto accidents, which are more frequent and, in some ways, more amenable to community control.

The determination to mount a major research effort to eradicate polio arose in no small part from the involvement of President Franklin D. Roosevelt, who was struck down by polio when a successful young politician. His determination to overcome his paralytic handicap and the commitment to the fight against polio made by Basil O'Connor, his former law partner, enabled a great deal of attention, effort, and money to be expended on the care and rehabilitation of polio victims and—in the end, more importantly—on research into the causes and prevention of the disease.

During the course of this research, it was discovered that polio is caused by a virus and that three main virus types are involved. Although clinical manifestations of polio are rare, it was discovered that the virus itself was not rare, but common, and that most adult individuals had experienced a polio infection sometime in their lives without ever being aware of it.

This finding helped to explain the otherwise peculiar circumstance that polio epidemics seemed to hit hardest those who were better off hygienically (i.e., those who had the best nutrition, most favorable housing conditions, and were otherwise apparently most favorably situated). Indeed, the disease seemed to be virtually unknown in those countries with the poorest hygiene. The explanation is that because there was plenty of polio virus in the less-favored populations, almost every infant was exposed to the disease early in life while he was still protected by the immunity passed on from his mother. As a result, everyone had had polio, but under protected circumstances, and, thereby, everyone had developed his own immunity.

As with many other virus diseases, an individual who has been infected by polio and recovered is usually immune to another attack (at least by a virus strain of the same type). The reason for this is that the body, in fighting the infection, develops *antibodies,* which are a part of the gamma globulin fraction of the blood, to the *antigen,* which is the protein part of the polio virus. These antibodies remain in the bloodstream for years, and even when their level declines so far as to be scarcely measurable, there are usually enough of them to prevent a serious attack from the same virus.

Smallpox and influenza illustrate two different approaches to the preparation of an effective vaccine. For smallpox, which has long been controlled by a vaccine, we use for the vaccine a closely related virus, cowpox, which is ordinarily incapable of causing serious disease in man, but which gives rise to antibodies that also protect against smallpox. (In a very few individuals this vaccine is capable of causing a severe, and occasionally fatal, reaction. The risk is small enough, however, so that we do not hesitate to expose all our school children to it in order to protect them from smallpox.) In the case of influenza, however, instead of a closely related live virus, the vaccine is a solution of the influenza virus itself, prepared with a virus that has been killed by treatment for a time with formaldehyde. Provided that the treatment is not too prolonged, the dead virus still has enough antigenic activity to produce the required antibodies so that, although it can no longer infect, it is, in this case, sufficiently like the live virus to be a satisfactory vaccine.

In the case of polio, both of these methods were explored. A live-virus vaccine would have the advantage of reproducing in the vaccinated individual and, hopefully, giving rise to a strong reaction which would produce a high level of long-lasting antibodies. With such a vaccine, however, there might be a risk that a vaccine virus so similar to the virulent polio virus could mutate into a virulent form and itself be the cause of paralytic or fatal disease. A killed-virus vaccine should be safe because it presumably could not infect, but it might fail to give rise to an adequate antibody response. These and other problems stood in the way of the rapid development of a successful vaccine. Some unfortunate prior experience also contributed to the cautious approach of researchers. In the thirties, attempts had been made to develop vaccines against polio; two of these were actually in use for a time. Evidence that at least one of these vaccines, in fact, had been responsible for cases of paralytic polio soon caused both to be promptly withdrawn from use. This experience was very much in the minds of polio researchers, and they had no wish to risk a repetition.

Research to develop both live and killed vaccines was stimulated in the late forties by the development of a tissue culture technique for growing polio virus. Those working with live preparations developed harmless strains from virulent ones by growing them for many generations in suitable tissue culture media. There was, of course, considerable worry lest these strains, when used as a vaccine in man, might revert to virulence and cause paralysis or death. (By 1972 it seems clear that the strains developed are indeed safe—a live-virus preparation taken orally is the vaccine presently in widespread use throughout the world.)

Those working with killed preparations, notably Jonas Salk, had the problem of treating the virus (with formaldehyde) sufficiently to eliminate its infectiousness, but not so long as to destroy its antigenic effect. This was more difficult than, at first, had appeared to be the case, and some early lots of the vaccine proved to contain live virus capable of causing paralysis and death. There are statistical issues in the safety story (Meier 1957), but our concern here is with the evaluation of effectiveness.

EVALUATION OF EFFECTIVENESS

In the early fifties the Advisory Committee convened by the National Foundation for Infantile Paralysis (NFIP) decided that the killed-virus vaccine developed by Jonas Salk at the University of Pittsburgh had been shown to be both safe and capable of inducing high levels of the antibody in children on whom it had been tested. This made the vaccine a promising candidate for general use, but it remained to prove that the vaccine actually would prevent polio in exposed individuals. It would be unjustified to release such a vaccine for general use without convincing proof of its effectiveness, so it was determined that a large-scale "field trial" should be undertaken.

That the trial had to be carried out on a very large scale is clear. For suppose we wanted the trial to be convincing if indeed the vaccine were 50% effective (for various reasons, 100% effectiveness could not be expected). Assume that, during the trial, the rate of occurrence of polio would be about 50 per 100,000 (which was about the average incidence in the United States during the fifties). With 40,000 in the control group and 40,000 in the vaccinated group, we would find about 20 control cases and about 10 vaccinated cases, and a difference of this magnitude could fairly easily be attributed to random variation. It would suggest that the vaccine might be effective, but it would not be persuasive. With 100,000 in each group, the expected numbers of polio cases would be 50 and 25, and such a result would be persuasive. In practice, a much larger study was clearly required, because it was important to get definitive results as soon as possible, and if there were relatively few cases of polio in the test area, the expected number of cases might be well under 40. It seemed likely, also, for reasons we shall discuss later, that paralytic polio, rather than all polio, would be a better criterion of disease, and only about half the diagnosed cases are classified "paralytic." Thus the relatively low incidence of the disease, and its great variability from place to place and time to time, required that the trial involve a huge number of subjects—as it turned out, over a million.

THE VITAL STATISTICS APPROACH

Many modern therapies and vaccines, including some of the most effective ones, such as smallpox vaccine, were introduced because preliminary studies suggested their value. Large-scale use subsequently provided clear evidence of efficacy. A natural and simple approach to the evaluation of the Salk vaccine would have been to distribute it as widely as possible, through the schools, to see whether the rate of reported polio was appreciably less than usual during the subsequent season. Alternatively, distribution might be limited to one or a few areas because limitations of supply would preclude effective coverage of the entire country. There is even a fairly good chance that were one to try out an effective vaccine against the common cold or against measles, convincing evidence might be obtained in this way.

In the case of polio—and, indeed, in most cases—so simple an approach would almost surely fail to produce clear cut evidence. First, and foremost, we must consider how much polio incidence varies from season to season, even without any attempts to modify it. From Figure 1, which shows the annual reported incidence from 1930 through 1955, we see that had a trial been conducted in this way in 1931, the drop in incidence from 1931 to 1932 would have been strongly suggestive of a highly effective vaccine because the incidence dropped to less than a third of its previous level. Similar misinterpretations would have been made in 1935, 1937, and other years—most recently in 1952. (On the general problem of drawing inferences from

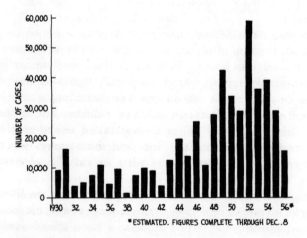

*ESTIMATED. FIGURES COMPLETE THROUGH DEC. 8

FIGURE 1

Poliomyelitis in the U.S., 1930–56. Source: Meier (1957)

such time series data see the essay by Campbell.) One might suppose that such mistakes could be avoided by using the vaccine in one area, say, New York State, and comparing the rate of incidence there with that of an unvaccinated area, say, Illinois. Unfortunately, an epidemic of polio might well occur in Chicago—as it did in 1956—during a season in which New York had a very low incidence.

Another problem, more subtle, but equally burdensome, relates to the vagaries of diagnosis and reporting. There is no difficulty, of course, in diagnosing the classic respirator case of polio, but the overwhelming majority of cases are less clearcut. Fever and weakness are common symptoms of many illnesses, including polio, and the distinction between weakness and slight transistory paralysis will be made differently by different observers. Thus the decision to diagnose a case as nonparalytic polio instead of some other disease may well be influenced by the physician's general knowledge or feeling about how widespread polio is in his community at the time.

These difficulties can be mitigated to some extent by setting down very precise criteria for diagnosis, but it is virtually impossible to obviate them completely when, as would be the case after the widespread introduction of a new vaccine, there is a marked shift in what the physician expects to find. This is most especially true when the initial diagnosis must be made by family physicians who cannot easily be indoctrinated in the use of a special set of criteria, as is the case with polio. Later evaluation by specialists cannot, of course, bring into the picture those cases originally diagnosed as something other than polio.

THE OBSERVED CONTROL APPROACH

The difficulties of the vital statistics approach were recognized by all concerned, and the initial study plan, although not judged entirely satisfactory, got around many of the problems by introducing a control group similar in characteristics to the vaccinated group. More specifically, the idea was to offer vaccination to all children in the second grade of participating schools and to follow the polio experience not only in these children, but in the first- and third-grade children as well. Thus the vaccinated second-graders would constitute the *treated* group, and the first- and third-graders would constitute the *control* group. This plan follows what we call the *observed control approach.*

It is clear that this plan avoids many of the difficulties that we listed above. The three grades all would be drawn from the same geographic location so that an epidemic affecting the second grade in a given school would certainly affect the first and third grades as well. Of course, all subjects would be observed concurrently in time. The grades, naturally, would be different ages, and polio incidence does vary with age. Not much variation from grade to grade was expected, however, so it seemed reasonable to assume that the average of first and third grades would provide a good control for the second grade.

Despite the relative attractiveness of this plan and its acceptance by the NFIP advisory committee, serious objections were raised by certain health departments that were expected to participate. In their judgment, the results of such a study were likely to be insufficiently convincing for two important reasons. One is the uncertainty in the diagnostic process mentioned earlier and its liability to influence by the physician's expectations, and the other is the selective effect of using volunteers.

Under the proposed study design, physicians in the study areas would have been aware of the fact that only second-graders were offered vaccine, and in making a diagnosis for any such child, they would naturally and properly have inquired whether he had or had not been vaccinated. Any tendency to decide a difficult diagnosis in favor of nonpolio when the child was known to have been vaccinated would have resulted in a spurious piece of evidence favoring the vaccine. Whether or not such an effect was really operating would have been almost impossible to judge with assurance, and the results, if favorable, would have been forever clouded by uncertainty.

A less conjectural difficulty lies in the difference between those families who volunteer their children for participation in such a trial and those who do not. Not at all surprisingly, it was later found that those who do volunteer tend to be better educated and, generally, more well-to-do than are those who do not participate. There was also evidence that those who agree to participate tend to be absent from school with a noticeably higher frequency than others. The direction of effect of such selection on the incidence of diagnosed polio is by no means clear before the fact, and this important difference between the treated group and the control group also would have clouded the interpretation of the results.

RANDOMIZATION AND THE PLACEBO CONTROL APPROACH

The position of critics of the NFIP plan was that the issue of vaccine effectiveness was far too important to be studied in a manner which would leave uncertainties in the minds of reasonable observers. No doubt, if the vaccine should appear to have fairly high effectiveness, most public health officials and the general public would accept it, despite the reservations. If, however, the observed control scheme were used, a number of qualified public health scientists would have remained unconvinced, and the value of the vaccine would be uncertain. Therefore, the critics proposed that the study be run as a scientific experiment with the use of appropriate randomizing procedures to assign subjects to treatment or to control and with a maximum effort to eliminate observer bias. This plan follows what we call the *placebo control approach.*

The chief objection to this plan was that parents of school children could not reasonably be expected to permit their children to participate in an experiment in which they might be getting only an ineffective salt solution instead of a probably helpful vaccine. It was argued further that the injection of placebo might not be ethically sound, since a placebo injection carries a small risk, especially if the child unknowingly is already infected with polio.

The proponents of the placebo control approach maintained that, if properly approached, parents *would* consent to their children's participation in such an experiment, and they judged that because the injections would not be given during the polio season, the risk associated with the placebo injection itself was vanishingly small. Certain health departments took a firm stand: they would participate in the trial only if it were such a well-designed experiment. The consequence was that in approximately half the areas, the randomized placebo control method was used, and in the remaining areas, the alternating-grade observed control method was used.

A major effort was put forth to eliminate any possibility of the placebo control results being contaminated by subtle observer biases. The only firm way to accomplish this was to insure that neither the subject, nor his parents, nor the diagnostic personnel could know which children had gotten the vaccine until all diagnostic decisions had been made. The method for achieving this result was to prepare placebo material that looked just like the vaccine, but was without any antigenic activity, so that the controls might be inoculated and otherwise treated in just the same fashion as were the vaccinated.

Each vial of injection fluid was identified only by a code number so that no one involved in the vaccination or the diagnostic evaluation process could know which children had gotten the vaccine. Because no one knew, no one could be influenced to diagnose differently for vaccinated cases and for controls. An experiment in which both the subject getting the treatment and the diagnosticians who will evaluate the outcome are kept in ignorance of the treatment given each individual is called a *double-blind* experiment. Experience in clinical research has shown the double-blind experiment to be the only satisfactory way to avoid potentially serious observer bias when the final evaluation is in part a matter of judgment.

For most of us, it is something of a shock to be told that competent and dedicated physicians must be kept in ignorance lest their judgments be colored by knowledge of treatment status. We should keep in mind that it is not deliberate distortion of findings by the physician which concern the medical experimenter. It is rather the extreme difficulty in many cases of making an uncertain decision which, experience has shown, leads the best of investigators to be subtly influenced by information of this kind. For example, in the study of drugs used to relieve postoperative pain, it has been found that it is quite impossible to get an unbiased judgment of the quality of pain relief, even from highly qualified investigators, unless the judge is kept in ignorance of which patients were given which drugs.

The second major feature of the experimental method was the assignment of subjects to treatments by a careful randomization procedure. As we observed earlier, the chance of coming down with a diagnosed case of polio varies with a great many factors including age, socioeconomic status, and the like. If we were to make a deliberate effort to match up the treatment and control groups as closely as possible, we should have to take care to balance these and many other factors, and, even so, we might miss some important ones. Therefore, perhaps surprisingly, we leave the balancing to a carefully applied equivalent of coin tossing: we arrange that each individual has an equal chance of getting vaccine or placebo, but we eliminate our own judgment entirely from the individual decision and leave the matter to chance.

The gain from doing this is twofold. First, a chance mechanism usually will do a good job of evening out all the variables—those we didn't recognize in advance, as well as those we did recognize. Second, if we use a chance mechanism in assigning treatments, we may be confident about the use of the theory of chance, that is to say, probability theory, to judge the results. We can then calculate the probability that so large a difference as that observed could reasonably be due solely to the way in which subjects were assigned to treatments, or whether, on the contrary, it is really an effect due to a true difference in treatments.

To be sure, there are situations in which a skilled experimenter can balance the groups more effectively than a random-selection procedure typically would. When some factors may have a large effect on the outcome of an experiment, it may be desirable, or even necessary, to use a more complex experimental design that takes account of these factors. However, if we intend to use probability theory to guide us in our judgment about the results, we can be confident about the accuracy of our conclusions only if we have used randomization at some appropriate level in the experimental design.

The final determinations of diagnosed polio proceeded along the following lines. First, all cases of poliolike illness reported by local physicians were subjected to special examination, and a report of history, symptoms, and laboratory findings was made. A special diagnostic group then evaluated each case and classified it as nonpolio, doubtful polio, or definite polio. The last group was subdivided into nonparalytic, paralytic, and fatal polio. Only after this process was complete was the code broken and identification made for each case as to whether vaccine or placebo had been administered.

RESULTS OF THE TRIAL

The main results are shown in Table 1, which shows the size of the study populations, the number of cases classified as polio, and the disease rates, that is, the number of cases per 100,000 population. For example, the second line shows that in the placebo control area there were 428 reported cases

TABLE 1. Summary of Study Cases by Diagnostic Class and Vaccination Status (Rates per 100,000)

STUDY GROUP	STUDY POPULATION	ALL REPORTED CASES		POLIOMYELITIS CASES								NOT POLIO	
		No.	Rate	Total		Paralytic		Nonparalytic		Fatal polio			
				No.	Rate	No.	Rate	No.	Rate	No.	Rate	No.	Rate
All areas: Total	1,829,916	1013	55	863	47	685	37	178	10	15	1	150	8
Placebo control areas: Total	749,236	428	57	358	48	270	36	88	12	4	1	70	9
Vaccinated	200,745	82	41	57	28	33	16	24	12	—	—	25	12
Placebo	201,229	162	81	142	71	115	57	27	13	4	2	20	10
Not inoculated*	338,778	182	54	157	46	121	36	36	11	—	—	25	7
Incomplete vaccinations	8,484	2	24	2	24	1	12	1	12	—	—	—	—
Observed control areas: Total	1,080,680	585	54	505	47	415	38	90	8	11	1	80	7
Vaccinated	221,998	76	34	56	25	38	17	18	8	—	—	20	9
Controls**	725,173	439	61	391	54	330	46	61	8	11	2	48	6
Grade 2 not inoculated	123,605	66	53	54	44	43	35	11	9	—	—	12	10
Incomplete vaccinations	9,904	4	40	4	40	4	40	—	—	—	—	—	—

Source: Adapted from Francis (1955), Tables 2 and 3.
* Includes 8,577 children who received one or two injections of placebo.
** First- and third-grade total population.

of which 358 were confirmed as polio, and among these, 270 were classified as paralytic (including 4 that were fatal). The third and fourth rows show corresponding entries for those who were vaccinated and those who received placebo, respectively. Beside each of these numbers is the corresponding rate. Using the simplest measure—all reported cases—the rate in the vaccinated group is seen to be half that in the control group (compare the boxed rates in Table 1) for the placebo control areas. This difference is greater than could reasonably be ascribed to chance, according to the appropriate probability calculation. The apparent effectiveness of the vaccine is more marked as we move from reported cases to paralytic cases to fatal cases, but the numbers are small and it would be unwise to make too much of the apparent, very high effectiveness in protecting against fatal cases. The main point is that the vaccine was a success; it demonstrated sufficient effectiveness in preventing serious polio to warrant its introduction as a standard public health procedure.

Not surprisingly, the observed control area provided results that were, in general, consistent with those found in the placebo control area. The volunteer effect discussed earlier, however, is clearly evident (note that the rates for those not innoculated differ from the rates for controls in both areas). Were the observed control information alone available, considerable doubt would have remained about the proper interpretation of the results.

Although there had been wide differences of opinion about the necessity or desirability of the placebo control design before, there was great satisfaction with the method after the event. The difference between the two groups, although substantial and definite, was not so large as to preclude doubts had there been no placebo controls. Indeed, there were many surprises in the more detailed data. It was known, for example, that some lots of vaccine had greater antigenic power than did others, and it might be supposed that they should have shown a greater protective effect. This was not the case; lots judged inferior in antigenic potency did just as well as those judged superior. Another surprise was the rather high frequency with which apparently typical cases of paralytic polio were not confirmed by laboratory test. Nonetheless, there were no surprises of a character to cast serious doubt on the main conclusion. The favorable reaction of those most expert in research on polio was expressed soon after the results were reported. By carrying out this kind of study before introducing the vaccine, it was noted, we now have facts about Salk vaccine that we still lack about typhoid vaccine, after 50 years of use, and about tuberculosis vaccine, after 30 years of use.

EPILOGUE

It would be pleasant to report an unblemished record of success for the Salk vaccine, following so expert and successful an appraisal of its effectiveness, but it is more realistic to recognize that such success is but one step in the continuing development of public health science.   The Salk vaccine, although a notable triumph in the battle against disease, was relatively crude and, in many ways, not a wholly satisfactory product that was soon replaced with better ones.

The report of the field trial was followed by widespread release of the vaccine for general use, and it was discovered very quickly that a few of these lots actually had caused serious cases of polio.   Distribution of the vaccine was then halted while the process was reevaluated.   Distribution was reinitiated a few months later, but the momentum of acceptance had been broken and the prompt disappearance of polio that researchers hoped for did not come about.   Meanwhile, research on a more highly purified killed-virus vaccine and on several live-virus vaccines progressed, and within a few years the Salk vaccine was displaced by live-virus vaccines.

The long-range historical test of the Salk vaccine, in consequence, has never been carried out.   We do not know with certainty whether or not that vaccine could have accomplished the relatively complete elimination of polio that has now been achieved.   Nonetheless, this does not diminish the importance of its role in providing the first heartening success in the attack on this disease, a role to which careful and statistically informed experimental design contributed greatly.

PROBLEMS

1. Using Figure 1 as an example, explain why a control group is needed in experiments where the effectiveness of a drug or vaccine is to be determined.

2. Explain the need for control groups by criticizing the following statement:
   "A study on the benefits of vitamin C showed that 90% of the people suffering from a cold who take vitamin C get over their cold within a week."

3. Explain the difference between the observed control approach and the placebo control approach. Which one would you prefer, and why?

4. Why is it important to have a "double-blind" experiment?

5. If "double-blind" experiments provide the only satisfactory way to avoid observer bias, why aren't they used all the time?

6. If only volunteers are used in an experiment, instead of a random sample of individuals, will the results of the experiment be of any value? What can you say about the results?

7. Why did the polio epidemics seem to hit hardest those who were better off hygienically?

8. Why was a *large-scale* field trial needed to get convincing evidence of the Salk vaccine effectiveness?

9. Refer to Figure 1. In which year did the highest polio incidence occur? the lowest? the largest increase? the smallest increase? Give the approximate values of these incidences and increases.

10. Refer to Figure 1. Comment on the use of the *number of cases*. Can you suggest a different indicator of the spread of poliomyelitis in the U.S. during 1930–56. When are the two indicators equivalent? (Hint: refer to Table 1.)

REFERENCES

K. Alexander Brownlee. 1955. "Statistics of the 1954 Polio Vaccine Trials." *Journal of the American Statistical Association* 50:272, pp. 1005–1013.

Thomas Francis, Jr., et al. 1955. "An Evaluation of the 1954 Poliomyelitis Vaccine Trials—Summary Report." *American Journal of Public Health* 45:5, pp. 1–63.

Paul Meier. 1957. "Safety Testing of Poliomyelitis Vaccine." *Science* 125:3257, pp. 1067–1071.

D. D. Rutstein. 1957. "How Good is Polio Vaccine?" *Atlantic Monthly* 199:48.

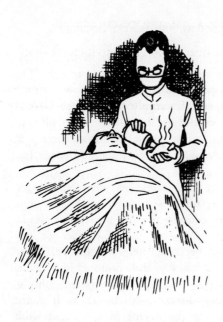

SAFETY OF ANESTHETICS

Lincoln E. Moses   *Stanford University*
Frederick Mosteller   *Harvard University*

In 1958, American hospitals began using a new anesthetic called halothane. It soon became widely accepted for its many desirable properties. Unlike some of the more commonly used anesthetics, it could not catch fire, so fire and explosive hazards did not have to be a concern during surgical operations. Patients found it less disagreeable and recovered from anesthesia more quickly and with less severe aftereffects. Extensive laboratory research and trials on animals and humans in surgery had encouraged belief in its safety. So there were good reasons for halothane to come rapidly into widespread use. By 1962, surgeons used halothane in half of their operations.

After a few years, however, halothane came under suspicion as accounts appeared in the medical literature of some strikingly unusual—but strikingly similar—deaths of patients who had recently had this anesthetic. A few patients recovering from surgery suddenly took a turn for the worse, ran fevers, and died; subsequent autopsies revealed massive fatal changes in their livers. Even though there were only a few such reports, it was natural to ask, "Do these incidents mean that halothane is a poison dangerous to people's livers? Should the use of halothane as an anesthetic in surgery therefore be discontinued?" Some compounds chemically similar to halothane were already known to cause liver damage, so the question arose with all the more force. A national committee was appointed to assemble and examine evidence that might help to answer these questions.

Much information was needed. First, it was possible that the liver changes found with halothane might occur equally often with other anesthetics, but that physicians rarely reported such cases because the old anesthetics would attract less attention. Second, and this is a key point, whether or not halothane had a special adverse effect on the liver, there was the possibility that its other advantages might result in a lower overall postoperative death rate. Frequently things that are easy to use actually work better (this is true of sharp knives, fine violins, and easy-to-read instructions), so it might well be that an anesthetic that is easier for the doctor to use might work better and result in somewhat lower death rates during surgery. Information was needed to confirm or refute this possibility.

These questions could not be answered by doing laboratory experiments with mice, for mice might well behave differently under the anesthetic than human beings; nor could the questions be answered by looking in books, for the information was not even known; nor was it useful to ask experts for their judgments, since different experts had widely different opinions.

THE EVIDENCE

It was necessary to amass a great deal of evidence, so the committee decided to conduct a survey of hospital experience. At that time, halothane had been given to about 10 million people in the U. S. Many of these patients had been in a particular group of 34 hospitals that kept good records and whose staffs keenly wanted to answer the very questions we have asked. They cooperated with the committee by sampling their records of surgical operations performed during the years 1960–64. In addition to recording whether or not the patient died within six weeks of surgery, they gave information on the anesthetic that had been used as well as facts about the surgical procedure and the patient's sex, age, and physical status prior to the operation. Among the 850,000 operations in the study, there were about 17,000 deaths, or a death rate of 2%. The death rates, shown in Table 1, were calculated for each of four major anesthetics and for a fifth group consisting of all other anesthetics. Note that these are death rates from all causes, including the patients' diseases, and are not deaths especially resulting from the anesthetic.

TABLE 1. Death Rates Associated with Various Anesthetics

HALOTHANE	PENTOTHAL*	CYCLOPROPANE	ETHER	ALL OTHER
1.7%	1.7%	3.4%	1.9%	3.0%

* Nitrous oxide plus barbiturate.

NEED FOR ADJUSTMENT

Table 1 suggests that halothane was as safe as any other anesthetic in wide use, but such a suggestion simply cannot be trusted. Medical people know that certain anesthetics, cyclopropane, for example, are used more often in severe and risky operations than some other anesthetics (such as pentothal, which is much less often used in difficult cases). So some or all of the differences between these death rates might be due to a tendency to use one anesthetic in difficult operations and another in easier ones.

Different operations carry very different risks of death. Indeed, death rates on some operations were found to be as low as 0.25% and on others nearly 14%. The change in death rates across the categories of patients' physical status was even more dramatic, ranging from 0.25% in the most favorable physical status category to over 30% in the least favorable. Age mattered a great deal: the most favorable 10-year age group (10 to 19) carried a death rate of less than 0.50%, while the least favorable age group (over 90) had a death rate of 26%. Another factor was sex, with women about two-thirds as likely to die. Because the factors of age, type of operation, physical status, and sex were so very important in determining the death rate, it was clear that even a relatively small preponderance of unfavorable patients in the group receiving a particular anesthetic could raise its death rate quite substantially. Thus, the differences in Table 1 *might* be due largely, and possibly even entirely, to discrepancies in the kinds of patients and types of operations associated with the various anesthetics. Certainly it was necessary to somehow adjust, to equalize for, type of operation, sex, physical status, and age before trying to determine the relative safety of the anesthetics.

If these data had been obtained from a properly planned experiment, the investigators might have arranged to collect the data so that patients receiving the various anesthetics were comparable in age, type of operation, sex, and physical status. As it was, these data were collected by reviewing old records, so substantial differences in the kinds of patients receiving the various anesthetics were to be expected and, indeed, were found. For example, cyclopropane was given two or three times more often than halothane to patients with bad physical status and substantially more often than halothane to patients over sixty years of age. There were many such peculiarities, and they were bound to affect the death rates of Table 1.

CARRYING OUT ADJUSTMENTS

The task was to purge the effects of these interfering variables from the death rates corresponding to the five anesthetics. Fortunately, it was possible to do this. We said "fortunately" because it could have been impossible; for example, if each anesthetic had been applied to a special set of operations, different from those in which other anesthetics were used, then differences found in the death rates could perfectly well have come from differences in the operations performed and there would be no way to disentangle operation from anesthetic and settle the question. But in the data of this study, there was much overlapping among the anesthetics in the categories of age, kind of operation, sex, and patient's physical status, so that statistical adjustment, or equalization, was possible. Analysis using such adjustment was undertaken in a variety of ways because the complexity of the problem made several different approaches reasonable and no one approach alone could be relied upon. There was close agreement in the findings regardless of the method used.

A summary of the results is shown in Table 2. Notice that halothane and pentothal after adjustment have higher death rates than their unadjusted rates in Table 1. Also, cyclopropane and "all other," the two with highest rates in Table 1, now have lower death rates. The effects of these adjustments are quite important: halothane, instead of appearing to be twice as safe as cyclopropane—the message in Table 1—now appears to be safer by only about one-fifth.

Figure 1 shows the adjustment effect graphically.

A Special, Simple Case. To understand the nature of the adjustments, it is helpful to look at a very special case with fictitious data.[1] Suppose that halothane and cyclopropane are to be compared, that we are to adjust only for physical status, and that we classify all patients in either good or poor physical

[1] This section may be skipped without disturbing continuity.

TABLE 2. Adjusted Death Rates for Various Anesthetics
(Adjusted for Age, Type of Operation, Sex, and Physical Status)

HALOTHANE	PENTOTHAL	CYCLOPROPANE	ETHER	ALL OTHER
2.1%	2.0%	2.6%	2.0%	2.5%

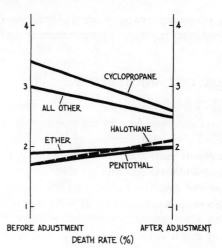

FIGURE 1
*Effects of adjusting death rates.
Plotted points are from Tables
1 and 2*

status. The fictitious data might look like those shown in Table 3. Thus, halothane was given to patients in good status four out of five times (in this fictitious case), but cyclopropane, just the other way around, was given to patients in good physical status one out of five times. The two anesthetics have exactly the same death rates for each physical status classification separately, but the very different proportions of status for the two make the overall death rate for cyclopropane almost twice that of halothane.

Suppose that we decide to adjust by computing what the overall death rates *would* be if the two anesthetics were given to a population of patients in which 70% were of good status and 30% poor. The death rates for each status group remain the same. The computations would be as displayed in Table 4. For each anesthetic the overall death rate is now 1.6% with these fictitious data.

TABLE 3.   Fictitious Data

	NUMBER OF PATIENTS	NUMBER OF DEATHS	DEATH RATE
Halothane			
Poor physical status	200	6	3.0%
Good physical status	800	8	1.0%
All patients	1000	14	1.4%
Cyclopropane			
Poor physical status	800	24	3.0%
Good physical status	200	2	1.0%
All patients	1000	26	2.6%

TABLE 4.   Adjusted Death Rates (Fictitious Data)

	NUMBER OF PATIENTS	NUMBER OF DEATHS	DEATH RATE
Halothane			
Poor physical status	300	9	3.0%
Good physical status	700	7	1.0%
All patients	1000	16	1.6%
Cyclopropane			
Poor physical status	300	9	3.0%
Good physical status	700	7	1.0%
All patients	1000	16	1.6%

In practice, the actual adjustments are far more complicated, partly because fine breakdowns of the data leave many cells with no entries at all and many with small entries.

Consistency over Hospitals.   Even after the adjustments, there was still considerable variability from hospital to hospital.   Our confidence in the validity of the statistically adjusted figures in Table 2 is affected by how consistent the death rates were from hospital to hospital.   After all, if there were many hospitals where cyclopropane had a lower adjusted death rate than did halothane, even though halothane was lower "on the average," we might feel uncertain that halothane was really safer just because of the difference in adjusted death rates.   Some fluctuation from hospital to hospital is to be expected, of course, because of chance factors; absolute consistency is not to be expected.

The question is: "Were the comparisons between the adjusted anesthetic death rates consistent enough over hospitals to warrant taking seriously the apparent differences shown in Table 2?"   Rather complicated statistical techniques were necessary to study this question, but the conclusions were clear: halothane and pentothal both had adjusted death rates definitely lower than the adjusted death rates for cyclopropane and "all other," and those lower adjusted death rates were real in the sense that they could not be explained by chance fluctuations.   The differences were sufficiently consistent to be believed.   On the other hand, ether, with the same adjusted death rate as halothane and pentothal, did not have a consistent pattern of comparison.   Therefore, ether cannot be reliably compared with the others; we cannot tell from the evidence obtained whether it may be somewhat safer than it appears here—or somewhat less safe.   Possibly it is as safe as, or safer than, halothane; possibly it is no safer than "all other."   The findings about ether are indefinite because there were fewer administrations of ether and these were concentrated in a few hospitals; hence there are fewer data to go on.

A SUMMING UP SO FAR

What can we conclude so far from the findings of this study? First, and most important, is the surprising result that halothane, which was suspect at the beginning of the study, emerged as a definitely safe and probably superior anesthetic agent. Second, we see that a careful statistical study of 850,000 operations enabled the medical profession to answer questions more firmly than had previously been possible, despite the much greater "experience" of 10 million administrations of halothane and other 10s of millions of administrations of the other anesthetics.

HOSPITAL DIFFERENCES AGAIN

A brand new question emerged with the observation that the 34 hospitals had very different overall postoperative death rates! These ranged from around 0.25% to around 6.5%. This seemed to mean that the likelihood of dying within six weeks after surgery could be more than 20 times as great in one hospital as in another. Just as before, however, there were strong reasons to approach this startling information skeptically. Some of the hospitals in the study did not undertake difficult operations, such as open-heart surgery, while others had quite large loads in such categories. This kind of difference alone would cause differences in hospital death rates. Further, the age distribution might be different, and perhaps importantly so, from one hospital to another. Indeed, one was a children's hospital, another a veteran's hospital. Some hospitals might more frequently accept surgical patients having poor physical status. So the same interfering variables as before surely affected the differences in hospital death rates. If adjustment was made for them, would the great differences in hospital death rates vanish? Be much reduced? Remain the same? Or, as is conceivable, actually increase?

Adjustment procedures were applied, and the result was that the high-death-rate hospitals, after adjustment, moved down toward a 2% overall death rate, and the low-death-rate hospitals, after adjustment, moved up toward a 2% overall death rate. The adjusted hospital death rates no longer ranged from 0.25% to over 6.5%; instead, the largest of these adjusted death rates was only about three times as great as the smallest. Now, almost any group of 34 such rates will exhibit some variability, and the ratio of the largest to the smallest must be a number larger than 1. Even if a single hospital were measured over several different periods, the rates would fluctuate from chance alone. The fluctuation in rate would be considerable because the death rate itself is basically low and one death more or less makes a difference in the observed rate for the period. The fact that this ratio turned out to be 3 in these data does not, in itself, indicate clearly that there were real, unexplained hospital differences.

Careful statistical study showed that there are probably some real differences from hospital to hospital in postoperative death rates, and that these differences cannot be explained wholly by the hospitals' patient populations in terms of age, sex, physical status, and surgical procedure. Statistical theory showed that the ratio of highest to lowest adjusted rate should be about 1.5 if the hospitals were identical in operative death rate after adjustment (so that the adjusted rates differ only by chance fluctuation).

The position, then, is that we began with the large ratio of about 25 for unadjusted rates, cut the ratio way down to 3 for adjusted rates, and then compared the 3 with 1.5 as a theoretical ratio. Because the adjustments can hardly have been perfect and because there undoubtedly were unadjusted factors that differed among the hospitals, we conclude that the adjusted hospital death rates are indeed close together. Thus, what, on the basis of the unadjusted hospital death rates, looked like a shocking public health problem proved, after statistical investigation, to be quite something else. The apparent problem was mainly, though perhaps not entirely, a dramatic manifestation of differences not in the quality of surgical care, but in the difficulty of the surgical cases handled in the various hospitals.

LIVER DAMAGE

Let us return to the question of liver damage. The total deaths from this source were few, and the lack of autopsies for nearly half of the deaths made firm conclusions impossible. Since the study was made, however, an anesthesiologist who had often been exposed to halothane while administering it to patients, has been discovered to be sensitive to halothane; he exhibits symptoms of liver malfunction from breathing it.

Are occasional individuals sensitive to other anesthetics? How many people develop such sensitivity? These are hard questions to answer, and they are especially difficult to study because of the rarity of the occurrences.

CONTRIBUTIONS OF STATISTICS

What were the main contributions of statistics in the program? First was the basic concept of a death-rate study. This needed to be carried out so that the safety of anesthetics could be seen in light of total surgical experience, not just in deaths from a single rare cause. Second, though we have not discussed it, the study used a special statistical technique of sampling records designed to save money and to produce a high quality of information. Third, special statistical adjustments had to be created to appraise the results when so many important variables—age, type of operation, sex, patient's physical status, and so on—were uncontrolled.   Fourth, as a result, the original premise of the study was not sustained, but a new result emerged: halothane seemed safer than cyclopropane.   The study produced a nonfact as well: the comparative merit of ether is uncertain.   We cannot tell if its associated death rate is higher, lower, or nearly the same as halothane, though the indication is that it is nearly the same.   Fifth, new evidence on hospital differences showed that the initial, wide variation in death rates, when suitably adjusted for patient populations, left only small unexplained differences in rates.   These remaining differences led the medical profession to begin, in 1971, a study of possible causes of hospital-to-hospital differences in postoperative death rates, in the hope of discovering ways to improve postoperative care.

PROBLEM

1. Explain how it was possible for halothane to be as safe as other anesthetics despite the evidence from autopsies that it caused liver damage.

2. What is meant by equalization or adjustment?

3. Explain the discrepancy between the safety of halothane indicated in Tables 1 and 2.

4. How can you explain the unadjusted differences of the overall postoperative death rates in the 34 hospitals in the study?

5. What were the principal conclusions of the study?

6. What statistical tools were used in the study?

7. Explain why the results about ether were uncertain.

8. Is halothane a cause of liver damage? Explain.

9. Refer to Figure 1. For which anesthetic is the adjustment most drastic? Check your answer by comparing Table 2 with Table 1.

10. In Table 4 explain how the number of deaths in each status group was calculated.

11. Consider a study of the effect of a high cholesterol diet on mortality from coronary heart disease. The mortality rates from CHD in two groups are compared—one group with high cholesterol diet and another with an average diet. What are some of the factors that one needs to adjust for in the two groups before comparing the mortality rates?

12. Why did the statistical study described in this article concentrate on 850,000 operations only although there were over 10 million operations in which halothane was administered and 10's of millions of operations where other anesthetics were used?

REFERENCE

John P. Bunker, William H. Forrest, Jr., Frederick Mosteller, and Leroy D. Vandam. 1969. *The National Halothane Study,* Report of the Subcommittee on the National Halothane Study of the Committee on Anesthesia, Division of Medical Sciences, National Academy of Sciences—National Research Council, published by the U. S. Government Printing Office, Washington, D. C., for the National Institutes of Health, National Institute of General Medical Sciences, Bethesda, Md.

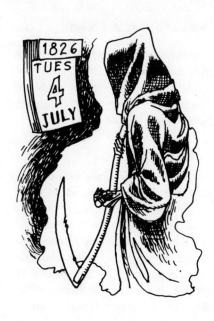

DEATHDAY AND BIRTHDAY:
An Unexpected Connection

David P. Phillips   *State University of New York, Stony Brook*

IN THE movies and in certain kinds of romantic literature, we sometimes come across a deathbed scene in which a dying person holds onto life until some special event has occurred. For example, a mother might stave off death until her long-absent son returns from the wars. Do such feats of will occur in real life as well as in fiction? If some people really do postpone death, how much can the timing of death be influenced by psychological, social, or other identifiable factors? Can deaths from certain diseases be postponed longer than deaths from other diseases?

In this essay we shall see how dying people react to one special event: their birthdays. We want to learn whether some people postpone their deaths until after their birthdays. If we compare the date of death with the date of birth for a large number of people, will we find fewer deaths than expected just before the birthday? If we do find a dip in deaths, we may conclude that some of these people are postponing death until after their birthdays.

We shall use elementary statistical methods in approaching the problem. For example, the comparison of an actual number of events with the number that might be expected is one of these methods; others will be noted later.

NATURE OF THE DATA TO BE INVESTIGATED

We shall examine only the deaths of famous people. There are two reasons for this. First, it seems likely that ordinary people look forward to their birthdays less eagerly than do famous people because a very famous person's birthday, generally, is celebrated publicly, and he may receive a substantial amount of attention, gifts, and so on. In contrast, much less attention is paid to the birthday of an ordinary person, and he may have relatively little reason to look forward to it. Hence famous people may be more likely to postpone deaths than less famous ones. Second, it is easier to examine the deaths of the famous than of other people. To discover whether there is a dip in deaths before the birthday, we need information on the birth and death dates of individuals. This type of information is not available from conventional tables of vital statistics; therefore, we cannot easily determine the birth and death dates of large numbers of ordinary people. On the other hand, we can easily determine the birth and death dates of famous people because there is much biographical information available about them.

In all, we shall examine the birth and death dates of more than 1200 people. It is tedious to classify these dates by *day,* so we shall examine the *month* of birth and *month* of death. Thus, for the purpose of this analysis, we shall be concerned, not with the relationship between the birthday and the day of death, but rather with the relationship between the birth month and the death month. For our purposes, a person is said to have died in his birth month if the month of his death has the same name as the month of his birth. For example, if a person was born on March 1, 1897, and died on March 31, 1950, he died in his birth month. On the other hand, if he was born on March 1 and died on February 28, he did not die in his birth month; rather, he died in the month just before his birth month. Although we gain convenience by examining events by month rather than by day, we lose precision; if we find a dip in deaths in the month before the birth month, we cannot tell whether a dying person is hanging on for a few days or for a few weeks.

IS THERE A DIP IN DEATHS BEFORE THE BIRTH MONTH?

Table 1 shows the month of birth and month of death of people listed in *Four Hundred Notable Americans.* For example, we can see from the first column that one person who was born in January died in January, two people who were born in January died in February, and so on. The column labeled "Row Total" gives the total number of people who died in each month and the row labeled "Column Total" gives the total number of people born in each month.

Table 1 enables us to compare two hypotheses. The first hypothesis states that the death month is related to (is dependent on) the birth month in that some people postpone death in order to witness their birthdays. This will be called the *death-dip hypothesis*. The second hypothesis states that no deaths are being postponed and that the month of death is not related to (is independent of) the month of birth. This will be called the *independence hypothesis*. (When we formulate our problem in terms of two hypotheses, one that we wish to disprove in order to lend credence to the other, and try to decide which hypothesis seems more consistent with the data, we are using a standard statistical testing procedure. The concept of "independence" is also an important part of many statistical hypotheses.)

Our general plan is to see whether the month immediately preceding the birth month has fewer deaths than the independence hypothesis suggests. As we explain below, it turns out that if the independence hypothesis were true, about $\frac{1}{12}$ of the deaths would occur in each of the six months preceding the birth month, $\frac{1}{12}$ in the birth month, and $\frac{1}{12}$ in each of the five following months. Although this may seem obvious, it actually depends upon detailed calculations because we must take into account that some calendar months produce more deaths than others and some produce more births than others. It is intuitively satisfying, nevertheless, that for the independence hypothesis, the calculations give nearly equal expected numbers of deaths for each of the twelve months preceding, during, and following the birth month.

We now compare the actual number of deaths before the birth month with the number of deaths that are expected, on the average, if the independence hypothesis is true. If the observed number of deaths is noticeably less than the expected number, there is a dip in deaths before the birth month.

First, we count the actual number of deaths in the month just before the birth month. If we sum the numbers in the starred cells in Table 1, we will have the total observed number of deaths in this period. This number is 16.

Now we calculate the total expected number of deaths in the month just before the birth month. If the independence hypothesis is true, then the death month is independent of the birth month. This means that the deaths of those born in any given month should be distributed throughout the year in the same way as the deaths of those born in any other month. Thus, because 6.32% [this is $(22/348) \times 100$] of all the deaths in Table 1 fall in December, 6.32% of those born in January should die in December, 6.32% of those born in February should die in December, and so on. In Table 1, we see that 11.2% [$39/348) \times 100$] of all deaths fall in April. Then,

TABLE 1. Number of Deaths by Month of Birth and Month of Death (Sample 1)

MONTH OF DEATH	MONTH OF BIRTH												ROW TOTAL
	Jan.	Feb.	Mar.	Apr.	May	June	July	Aug.	Sept.	Oct.	Nov.	Dec.	
Jan.	1*	1*	2	1	2	2	4	3	1	4	2	4	27
Feb.	2	3	1*	3	1	0	2	1	2	2	6	4	27
Mar.	5	6	5	3*	1	0	5	1	2	5	3	1	37
Apr.	7	6	3	2	1*	3	3	1	3	2	4	4	39
May	4	4	2	2	1	2*	4	1	2	2	1	5	31
June	4	0	4	5	2	1	1*	2	1	2	4	0	25
July	4	0	3	4	3	3	4	1*	6	4	2	5	39
Aug.	4	4	4	4	2	2	3	3	1*	1	2	0	30
Sept.	2	2	1	0	2	0	2	4	2	0*	5	2	22
Oct.	4	2	2	3	2	2	2	3	3	1	4*	5	33
Nov.	0	2	0	2	1	1	0	3	3	3	1	0*	16
Dec.	1*	2	2	1	2	1	4	1	4	0	2	2	22
COLUMN TOTAL	38	32	29	30	19	17	34	24	31	26	36	32	
TOTAL													348†

Source: R. B. Morris, ed., *Four Hundred Notable Americans* (New York: Harper & Row, 1965).
* Deaths corresponding to month preceding birth month.
† The total number of deaths is less than 400 because (1) some of those in the volume have not yet died; (2) for some of those in the volume, the month of birth and/or death is not known.

if independence holds, we would expect 11.2% of those born in any month to die in April. For example, there are 19 people born in May; we expect 11.2% of these people, that is, $(11.2/100) \times 19 = 2.1$, to die in April. In a similar fashion, we can work out the expected number of deaths in each of the 12 starred cells in Table 1. If we sum these 12 numbers, we will have the total number of deaths that we expect to occur in the month before the birth month *if* the independence hypothesis is true. This expected number is 28.3.

The more intuitive method mentioned earlier estimates the total expected number of deaths in the starred cells to be simply $348/12 = 29.0$. In other words, we expect about $\frac{1}{12}$ of all deaths to occur one month before the birth month. In fact, we expect about $\frac{1}{12}$ of all deaths to occur in the birth month or in any month before or after it. In general, this rough-and-ready method of estimating the total expected number for any month gives results very close to those provided by more precise methods.

We can now compare the observed number of deaths before the birth month with the expected number in this period. No matter which "expected number" we use, it is considerably higher than the number of deaths observed just before the birth month: we expect about 28 or 29 deaths, but we observe only 16—about 12 fewer than expected. In other words, we observe a dip in deaths in the month before the birth month as predicted by the death-dip hypothesis. As we shall soon see, the discrepancy is much more than might reasonably be explained by chance.

IS THERE A DEATH RISE AFTER THE BIRTH MONTH?

If the death-dip hypothesis is true, what will become of the 12 or so people who presumably have postponed death until their birthdays? When are they expected to die? There is no way of answering this question a priori because, even if the death-dip hypothesis is true, the death dip might have come about in a number of different ways; some of these different ways imply differing periods of survival for those who have postponed death. For example, the death dip could result entirely because some people who were hovering between life and death unexpectedly recovered; in this case, it might be years before these people die, and we could expect no rise in deaths immediately after the birth month. On the other hand, the death dip could appear solely because those who do not die just before their birthdays live a few days or weeks longer than expected; in this case, there should be a peak in deaths soon after the birth month. Depending on the way in which the death dip came about, we would or would not expect a rise in deaths after the birth month: we cannot tell what to expect on the basis of the death-dip hypothesis.

Although the death-dip hypothesis is not helpful here, practical experience with another sample (of famous Englishmen) suggests that we look for a rise in deaths in the four-month period consisting of the birth month and the three months thereafter. Thus, although we searched for a *death dip* in a *one-month* period, we shall search for a *death rise* in a *four-month* period, because past experience, not theory, makes this approach seem promising.

Table 2 gives the observed number of deaths six months before the birth month, five months before, and so on, down to zero months before, one month after, and so on up to five months after the birth month. Because $n = 348$ is the total number of people in sample 1, $n/12 = 29.0$ is the number expected to die six months before the birth month, five months before, and so on. From this table it is evident that not only is there a dip in deaths before the birth month, but there is also a rise in deaths during the birth month and during the three months thereafter. We expect about $\frac{4}{12}$ of all deaths in the first sample [$348 \times (\frac{4}{12}) = 116$] to fall in this four-month period, but we observe 140 deaths during this time.

COULD THE DEATH DIP AND DEATH RISE BE DUE TO CHANCE?

We know that surprising phenomena sometimes occur just by chance and for no other reason. For example, a person might deal himself a straight in poker; ordinarily, we attribute this happy event to the vagaries of providence, not to the dishonesty of the dealer. In much the same way, we might wonder whether the death dip and death rise have arisen by chance and for no other reason.

Now suppose our poker player were to deal himself not just one straight, but four straights in a row in the four times he deals while playing with us. This *could* have happened by chance, but it is so unlikely that we would prefer some other explanation. The less likely an event is to occur by chance, the more we prefer some other explanation. Similarly, if we find a death dip and death rise in, say, four samples and not just one, there is a small possibility that these phenomena could have occurred by chance, but another explanation might be more plausible.

In sample 1 we observed that there are fewer deaths than expected in the month before the birth month, and more deaths than expected in the four-month period consisting of the birth month and the three months there-after. Can we find a similar death dip and death rise in other samples of people?

MORTALITY IN THREE MORE SAMPLES

Three new samples were taken, consisting of people who are famous for two reasons. First, they achieved high status in their lifetimes: they were listed in *Who Was Who in America*. Second, they came from well-known families (e.g., Adams, Vanderbilt, Rockefeller) which are listed in "The Fore-most Families of the U.S.A.," an appendix to *Royalty, Peerage and Aristocracy*

TABLE 2. Number of Deaths, Before, During, and After the Birth Month (Sample 1)

	6 MONTHS BEFORE	5 MONTHS BEFORE	4 MONTHS BEFORE	3 MONTHS BEFORE	2 MONTHS BEFORE	1 MONTH BEFORE	THE BIRTH MONTH	1 MONTH AFTER	2 MONTHS AFTER	3 MONTHS AFTER	4 MONTHS AFTER	5 MONTHS AFTER
NUMBER OF DEATHS	24	31	20	23	34	16	26	36	37	41	26	34

$n = 348$
$n/12 = 29.0$

Source: Table 1.

of the World (vol. 90, 1967). We have ensured that the new samples do not overlap each other or sample 1.

Three volumes of *Who Was Who* were examined, those for the years 1951–60, 1943–50, and 1897–1942. Sample 2 contains all who are listed in the first of these volumes and have their surnames in "Foremost Families." Sample 3 contains all who are listed in the second *Who Was Who* volume and have their surnames in "Foremost Families." Sample 4 contains *every other* person who is in the third volume of *Who Was Who* and has his surname in "Foremost Families." We chose every other person rather than every person because the third volume is so much larger than the other volumes that it would be tedious to examine every person who meets our selection criteria.

Table 3 gives the observed number of deaths before, during, and after the birth month for samples 2, 3, and 4. The last number in each row of this table is the expected number of deaths six months before the birth month, five months before, and so on. We can see that the death dip and death rise evident in sample 1 also appear in samples 2, 3, and 4. In each of these samples there are fewer deaths than expected in the month before the birth month and more deaths than expected in the four-month period consisting of the birth month and the three months thereafter.

If we now combine the data in all four samples, we get the results seen in Table 4. A graph of these results appears in Figure 1, where we can see a death dip just before the birth month and a death rise during and after it.

In summary, just before the birth month, in each of the four samples presented, we found fewer deaths than would be expected under the hypothesis that the month of death is independent of the month of birth. In each of the four samples presented, more deaths occur during and immediately after the birth month than would be expected if independence held. The similarity of results in each of the four samples helps to convince us that the death dip and death rise are real phenomena and are not merely chance fluctuations in the data.

THE SIZE OF THE DEATH DIP AND DEATH RISE

Let us estimate the size of the death dip before the birth month and the size of the death rise thereafter for the aggregate sample of 1251 people. Out of 1251 people, 86 died in the month before the birth month. Given independence between the birth month and the death month, we would expect about $\frac{1}{12}$ of all 1251 deaths, or approximately 104 deaths, to fall in this period. Thus, just before the birth month only about 83% (86/104) of the deaths expected actually occurred. To put this another way, in the month before the birth month there were about 17% fewer deaths than we would expect under independence.

Table 3. Number of Deaths Before, During, and After the Birth Month Samples 2, 3, and 4

NUMBER OF DEATHS	6 MONTHS BEFORE	5 MONTHS BEFORE	4 MONTHS BEFORE	3 MONTHS BEFORE	2 MONTHS BEFORE	1 MONTH BEFORE	THE BIRTH MONTH	1 MONTH AFTER	2 MONTHS AFTER	3 MONTHS AFTER	4 MONTHS AFTER	5 MONTHS AFTER	TOTAL	TOTAL / 12
Sample 2*	17	23	26	27	28	28	42	32	31	34	36	30	354	29.5
Sample 3†	10	14	12	11	8	12	15	15	15	13	20	13	158	13.2
Sample 4‡	39	32	29	35	31	30	36	35	38	26	31	29	391	32.6

* Sample 2 excludes those listed in *Who Was Who in America 1951–1960* who died outside of that period and those listed in *Four Hundred Notable Americans*.
† Sample 3 excludes those listed in *Who Was Who in America 1943–1950* who died outside of that period or during World War II and those listed in *Four Hundred Notable Americans*.
‡ Sample 4 excludes those listed in *Who Was Who in America 1897–1942* who died outside of that period or during both World Wars and those listed in *Four Hundred Notable Americans*.

TABLE 4. Number of Deaths Before, During, and After the Birth Month, (All Samples Combined)

	6 MONTHS BEFORE	5 MONTHS BEFORE	4 MONTHS BEFORE	3 MONTHS BEFORE	2 MONTHS BEFORE	1 MONTH BEFORE	THE BIRTH MONTH	1 MONTH AFTER	2 MONTHS AFTER	3 MONTHS AFTER	4 MONTHS AFTER	5 MONTHS AFTER
NUMBER OF DEATHS	90	100	87	96	101	86	119	118	121	114	113	106

$n = 1251$
$n/12 = 104.3$

120

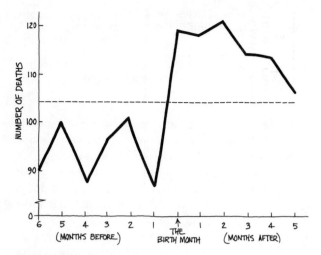

FIGURE 1

Number of deaths before, during, and after birth month (all samples combined)

Similarly, we can estimate the size of the death rise during the birth month and the three months thereafter.   There were 472 deaths in the period including the birth month and one, two, and three months thereafter.   Given independence between birth and death months, the expected number of deaths in this four-month period is estimated to be $\frac{4}{12}$ of all deaths, or 417 deaths $[(\frac{4}{12}) \times 1251 = 417]$.   Thus the actual number of deaths in and just after the birth month is $\frac{472}{417} = 11\%$ more than the number expected.

We can see that the death dip and death rise for sample 1 are larger than the death dips and death rises for the other three samples examined.   In the month before the birth month, sample 1 has 45% fewer deaths than independence leads us to expect.   In the remaining three samples combined, we observe 70 deaths in the month before the birth month; given independence, we expect about 75.25 $[(\frac{1}{12}) \times 903]$ in this period.   Thus, just before the birth month, the observed number of deaths in samples 2, 3, and 4 combined is approximately 7% less than the number expected under independence.

Similarly, it is evident that the death rise in sample 1 is larger than the death rises in the remaining samples.   We estimate that in sample 1, in the birth month and in the three months thereafter, there are 20% more deaths than expected.   The equivalent figure for samples 2, 3, and 4 is 10%.

The death dip and death rise in the sample 1 may be larger than in the other samples because the members of sample 1 are considerably more famous than the members of the other samples.   The 348 people in sample

1 are supposed to be the most famous people in American history. The larger number of people in the remaining samples were less stringently selected.

RELATION BETWEEN FAME AND THE SIZE OF THE DEATH DIP AND DEATH RISE

We have referred several times to the notion that a group of famous people is expected to produce a larger death dip before the birth month than a group of ordinary people. Now we shall assess this idea more carefully. We classify the members of sample 1 into three groups according to how famous they are and examine the sizes of the death dip and death rise produced by each of these groups. If we are right, we should find that the more famous a group is, the larger its death dip and death rise.

There are obviously many ways to classify groups by fame. The method used here is convenient and seems plausible. The best-known members of "the four hundred" are those whose names have become household words in the "common culture." The "common culture" may be said to consist of the knowledge shared by almost all the members of a society—in other words, some sort of lowest common denominator of knowledge. To find which of the four hundred is "in" the common culture, we must find a set of people who know only what is in that culture. The members of the four hundred who are known to this group of people have names that are part of the common culture.

Of all the people in a society, children come closest to having no more knowledge than is in the common culture. If a child has heard of someone in the four hundred, he is very famous indeed. Thus the members of the four hundred who appear in children's biographies may be judged to be better known than members who do not appear in such biographies.

Two series of children's biographies were examined: Dodd, Mead's (1966) and Bobbs-Merrill's (1966). The criterion of coverage or noncoverage in these series can be used to classify members of the four hundred into groups of differing fame. Three different subgroups were formed from the original four hundred.

Group 1 consists of those of the four hundred whose names are found in both of the children's biography series. For example, George Washington, Thomas Jefferson, Benjamin Franklin, Mark Twain, and Thomas Edison are in group 1.

Group 2 consists of those of the four hundred whose names are in only one of the series. For example, John Quincy Adams, John Hancock, Jefferson Davis, Edgar Allen Poe, and Alexander Graham Bell are in group 2.

Group 3 consists of those of the four hundred whose names are in neither series. For example, Samuel Adams, Millard Fillmore, Rutherford B. Hayes, H. L. Mencken, and Nikola Tesla are in group 3.

For our purposes, the members of group 1 are judged to be more famous, on the average, than the members of group 2, and the members of group 2 are judged to be more famous, on the average, than the members of group 3. We say "on the average" because single individuals could be moved readily from one group to another if we used a third or fourth biography series to judge fame. But we think that the groups as a whole are ordered with respect to fame in the way we want them to be.

We can now measure the death dip and death rise produced by each of these groups. Table 5 gives the relevant information.

As predicted, the more famous a group is, the larger is its death dip. Group 1 produces a larger death dip than group 2, and group 2 produces a larger death dip than group 3. The death dip for the most famous group is quite large. About 78% of the deaths that are expected to fall in the month before the birth month do not do so. It should be stressed, however, that the number of people in group 1 is not large.

From Table 5 we can see also that the more famous the group is, the larger is the death rise that it produces. In group 1 (the most famous group) the observed number of deaths during and just after the birth month is about 58% greater than the number expected. Note that there is no death rise at all for group 3, the least famous group.

SUMMARY

We have noted two sets of findings that are consistent with the notion that some people postpone death to witness a birthday because it is important to them. There is a death dip before the birth month and a death rise thereafter in four separate samples. We have noted also a consistent relation

TABLE 5.   The Size of the Death Dip and Death Rise for Groups of Differing Fame

GROUP	SIZE OF DEATH DIP (%)	SIZE OF DEATH RISE (%)	TOTAL NO. IN GROUP	NO. OF DEATHS IN THE BIRTH MONTH, AND 1, 2, 3 MONTHS THEREAFTER	NO. OF DEATHS IN THE MONTH BEFORE THE BIRTH MONTH
1	−78	58	55	29	1
2	−63	23	129	53	4
3	−20	−3	164	53	11

between the fame of a group and the size of its death dip and death rise: the more famous the group, the larger the death dip and death rise it produces. These results might be due to chance, but this possibility is sufficiently small that we would prefer some other explanation of these phenomena.

There are indications that some people postpone dying in order to witness events other than their birthdays. There are fewer deaths than expected before the Jewish Day of Atonement in New York, a city with a large Jewish population. In addition, there is a dip in U.S. deaths, in general, before U.S. Presidential elections.

We have anecdotal evidence that the timing of death might be related to other important social events. For example, many people have noted that both Jefferson and Adams died on July 4th, 50 years after the Declaration of Independence was signed. We may find it easier to believe that this is not coincidental if we read Jefferson's last words, quoted by his physician.[1]

> About seven o'clock of the evening of that day, he [Jefferson] awoke, and seeing my staying at his bedside exclaimed, "Oh Doctor, are you still there?" in a voice however, that was husky and indistinct. He then asked, "Is it the Fourth?" to which I replied, "It soon will be." These were the last words I heard him utter.

PROBLEMS

1. Why does the article examine the deaths of famous people only?

2. State and describe the two hypotheses being tested.

3. For the data in Table 1 is the assumption that "1/12 of the deaths occur each month" reasonable? Give reasons.

4. Calculate the expected number of deaths in each of the twelve starred cells in Table 1 under the assumption of independence, using the first method described in the text. Check that the expected total number of deaths in the month before the birth month is 28.3.

5. When would the two methods of estimating the total expected number of deaths in the month just before the birth month give exactly the same answer?

6. Refer to Figure 1.

   a. What is the meaning of the dotted line?

   b. Read from the graph the approximate number of deaths 1.5 months before the birth month. Is this figure meaningful? Why or why not?

---

[1] Merrill Peterson, *Thomas Jefferson and the New Nation* (New York: Oxford University Press, 1970), p. 1008.

c. Suppose that the death month of famous people is really independent of the birth month. Would you then expect the graph to be a horizontal line? Why or why not?

7. Consider the following alternative explanation (which might be called the birthday bash theory) for the death rise during and after the birth month:

"The reason for a death rise during these specific months is that famous people tend to exhaust themselves during the heavy celebrations on their birthdays thereby increasing the chance of death shortly after that date."

From the data presented in this article can one distinguish between this explanation and the one proposed in the article?

8. Do you think sample 4 is an appropriate sample of the people whose names appear in the 1897–1942 volume of "Who Was Who" and whose surnames appear in "Foremost Families"? Comment.

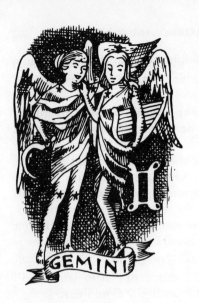

DOES INHERITANCE MATTER IN DISEASE?
THE USE OF TWIN STUDIES IN
MEDICAL RESEARCH

D. D. Reid   *London School of Hygiene and Tropical Medicine*

THE CONTROVERSY about the relative importance of nature and nurture that goes on in fields such as psychology also goes on in medicine. The crucial question is "Do we go mad or develop heart disease because we inherit a special susceptibility to a disease from our parents, or are these diseases the result of a stressful environment throughout our lives?" With most diseases, we cannot decide because patients almost always differ in both their nature, or genetic endowment, and their nurture, or environment, during the formative years of childhood, and of course, both can be important in particular diseases. Yet it is important to know whether in coronary heart disease, for example, it is worth persuading a patient to alter his environment by stopping smoking. If he both smokes heavily and has heart disease because he has inherited an anxious, worrying temperament, then altering his smoking habit alone might have disappointingly little effect. For these reasons, medical research in this area has concentrated on the unique and unusual opportunities presented by the occurrence of disease in twins.

The idea for this approach came from the English biometrician Francis Galton in 1875. He pointed out that there are two kinds of twins, identical and nonidentical. Identical twins come from the same fertilized egg and therefore have the same set of genes, which determine their physical and mental characteristics. Nonidentical twins, like ordinary siblings born at different times, come from separate eggs and their gene patterns are no more (and no less) alike than those of ordinary brothers and sisters (see Figure 1). Both types of twins, however, usually share the same family environment during their childhood and are usually treated alike by their parents. If, then, one of the pair develops a disease that is transmitted through the genes, it is more likely to appear in his identical twin than in a twin who is genetically different. On the other hand, in diseases due to diet or some other aspect of family life that is not genetically determined in the strict sense, the identical and nonidentical twin siblings of affected children are equally likely to develop the disease. Thus, we can get some indication of the relative importance of heredity and environment in causing a specific disease by comparing the

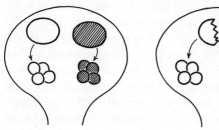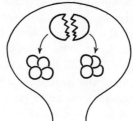

FIGURE 1

Genes determining light hair are indicated (O) and dark hair (●). Nonidentical twins come from separate eggs which carry different genetic elements that determine color of hair in the two children. It may or may not be different in the case of nonidentical twins. Part (a) illustrates an instance in which hair color is different. Identical twins result from the division of the same egg and so retain the same genetic element. Both children thus have the same hair color

TABLE 1.   Concordance Example
(O = Unaffected; ⊙ = Affected)

PAIR NUMBER	FIRST TWIN	SECOND TWIN
1	⊙	⊙
2	⊙	⊙
3	⊙	⊙
4	⊙	⊙
5	⊙	O
6	⊙	O

relative risk of the twin being affected when they are identical twins to that risk when they are nonidentical.   The difference in risk will be high in diseases where inheritance is important and low where it is not.

MEASURES OF DISEASE "CONCORDANCE"

These risks of the coincidence of disease appearing in both twins are measured in two ways.   Both methods aim to assess the degree of *concordance*, or agreement, between the disease experience of identical and nonidentical twins. Table 1 is a model population of six sets of identical twins.   One measure of the risk of both being affected is the "pair-wise concordance rate."   In this example, in four out of the six pairs, both twins are affected, so the "pair-wise concordance rate" is $4/6 \times 100\%$ or $66\frac{2}{3}\%$.   Pairs in which neither twin has the disease do not enter this diagram.   The second measure depends on the relative frequency or risk of the twin of an affected person also suffering from the disease.   This "proband concordance rate," or "affected concordance rate," in the example is given by the ratio of the number of twins affected as pairs (8) to the total number of affected people (10), that is, $8/10$ or 80%.   The "affected concordance rate" is perhaps the more widely used in twin studies.   (Knowing one of these measures, we can readily obtain the other, so no important choice is being made here; it is more a question of custom.)

SOME RESULTS FROM THE DANISH TWIN REGISTRY

Table 2 compares the "affected concordance rates" for identical and nonidentical pairs of Danish twins of whom at least one is affected by one of the diseases listed.   The high rates in identical twins versus the lower ones for nonidentical twins for tuberculosis (54 versus 27), rheumatoid arthritis (50 versus 5), bronchial asthma (63 versus 38), and epilepsy (54 versus 24) suggest a strong genetic element in these diseases.   On the other hand, death

TABLE 2. Occurrence of Selected Somatic Diseases in the Danish Twin Register Based on a Survey of 4368 Same-Sexed Pairs

DISEASE	AFFECTED CONCORDANCE RATES (%)			
	Identical Rate	No.*	Nonidentical Rate	No.*
Cerebral apoplexy	36	120	19	164
Coronary occlusion	33	122	27	179
Tuberculosis	54	185	27	309
Rheumatic fever	33	178	10	238
Rheumatoid arthritis	50	63	5	73
Death from acute infection	14	137	11	235
Bronchial asthma	63	94	38	125
Epilepsy	54	37	24	49

* Numbers refer to number of affected individuals, not pairs.

from acute infections other than tuberculosis and rheumatic fever (14 versus 11) shows no such disparity between the identical and nonidentical pairs of twins. Chance exposure to infection, perhaps outside the home, seems, therefore, to be much more important than any inherited susceptibility.

THE UNUSUALNESS OF TWINS

These examples have shown the potential of this method of distinguishing between genetic and environmental factors in different diseases. A word of caution is needed, however, about the risks of generalizing from the twins to the population as a whole, for twins are unusual in more senses than one. They are unusual in that multiple births occur relatively infrequently. A recent survey in the U.S. has shown that the proportion of twins has been falling in recent years. In 1964, 1 in 96 deliveries were of twins. (Triplets and quadruplets occurred once in 9977 and once in 663,470 deliveries— compared with the ratios of 1 in 9216 and 1 in 884,730 expected on the basis of the Helin–Zeleny hypothesis, that is, if twins occur once in 96 deliveries, triplets and quadruplets will occur once in 96×96 deliveries and $96 \times 96 \times 96$ deliveries respectively. It does not concern us here.)

Most important from the medical point of view is the fact that twins are more likely to be born to black than to white Americans and especially to older mothers who have already had several children. In a condition like mongolism, which is particularly common in children born to older women who have had large families, twins are thus likely to be more often affected than are singletons. Because twins have to depend on nutrients designed for a single child in the womb, they start at a disadvantage and are more likely to be born prematurely and to have difficult births. It is hardly surprising that their death rate in infancy and early childhood is higher than average. As they grow older, their disadvantage lessens, and in respect to the diseases of adult life, their experience is probably close to that of singletons. Thus, assessments based on observing disease in middle-aged twins are likely to be reasonably applicable to people in general.

PRACTICAL ASPECTS OF TWIN STUDIES

Sampling Populations of Twins. Early studies of disease in twins were often based on the patient with an unusual disease who came to the hospital and was found to have a twin suffering from the same condition. As in clinical medicine in general, the apparently unusual tends to be noted and published. Series of such coincidences in twins have thus been given prominence in the medical literature. But, because of the haphazard method of collection, such series are unlikely to give a true picture of the incidence of disease in the population of twins as a whole. Volunteer series, recruited perhaps by appeals in press or radio, are also likely to be biased. The ideal is to collect information either on all twins born in a generation or at least on a randomly selected, and thus truly representative, sample of them. Particularly in Scandinavia where vital records have long been accurate and complete, national twin registers have been established on this basis to serve medical and social research.

Some results from the Danish Twin Register have already been given. This Register comprised all twins born in Denmark during a defined period (1870–1910). Of the 37,914 twin births that occurred during that time, over half of the pairs had been broken by the death of one or both twins before their sixth birthday; these were not followed up. About 40% of the pairs were of different sex and not so useful for investigating diseases occurring in one sex more than another. Of the remainder, some 60% were nonidentical twins of the same sex and 40% identical and so like-sexed pairs. (In other words, the elimination of mixed-sex pairs from the surviving sets of twins changed the identical-nonidentical ratio of twin births from the usual 20:80 to 40:60.)

Establishing Type of Twins. Having identified and traced the twins through the population registers and other means, a problem arises in establishing their type by methods that can be widely and simply applied. In studies of small numbers, refined techniques can be used to compare inherited characteristics such as blood groups or blood-protein patterns to see whether in all such respects twins are truly identical. Fingerprints, voice sounds, and other physical traits can also be used. For large scale surveys in which subjects cannot be examined, but only interrogated by postal questionnaires, simpler methods are needed. It is fortunate, therefore, that the reply to one question is surprisingly effective in distinguishing identical from nonidentical pairs of twins. That question may take the form of "Were you as like as two peas in a pod?" and it is encouraging to note that when this question indeed was asked, over 95% of pairs in which both answered "yes" proved, on blood and other examination, to be identical, and when both answered "no," over 95% were fraternal; finally, 2% disagreed.

Once the pairs of twins have been classified, their disease experience must be ascertained. This can be done by collecting hospital records or death certificates over a period of years or by asking questions directly about either past illnesses or the presence of symptoms of chronic diseases such as coronary heart disease or rheumatism.

Other Applications of Twin Studies. Twin studies also may help to detect the effects of environmental factors in disease. Cigarette smoking, for example, is believed to cause other lung diseases as well as lung cancer. As in the case of lung cancer, it could be argued that an individual inherits both a liability to take up smoking and a specific susceptibility to lung diseases such as chronic bronchitis. If this were true, the apparent association between cigarette smoking and the presence of bronchitis could be dismissed as an effect arising at least in part from other causes rather than as proof that smoking caused bronchitis.

Surveys of smoking habits in identical and nonidentical twins have shown that there is indeed some evidence of a genetic element that affects smoking habit. Regarding smoking as a disease, we can, as before, compare the affected-concordance rate" in identical sets of twins with that in nonidentical sets. This shows that, if one of a set of twins smokes, his twin is more likely also to be a smoker if he is an identical twin than if he is a fraternal twin and, thus, no more closely related than an ordinary brother.

Because of this genetic element in smoking, the independent effect of smoking on bronchitis has to be assessed by comparing the frequency of bronchitis in identical twins who share the same genetic endowment but smoke different amounts. A survey based on the Swedish National Twin Study has done just this and the results for both types of twin are given in Table 3. These are set out simply in the form of prevalence rates which give the percentage of people in each twin and smoking group who have chronic coughs. Clearly, within each group of identical twins, smokers have higher prevalence rates for chronic cough than nonsmokers. In other words, even when the genetic background is identical, smoking appears to be associated with more bronchitis and thus is likely to be its cause.

Related Ideas. The use of twins is not confined to studies of medicine or biology; they have been used in studies of reading, for example. The idea of using identical twins as a control in the smoking investigation is a special

Table 3.   Prevalence of Cough Among Smokers and
Nonsmokers in Smoking Discordant Twin Pairs

	COUGH PREVALENCE (%)		TOTAL NUMBER OF CASES
	Smokers	Nonsmokers	
Identical twins			
Men	14.6	7.7	274
Women	13.6	7.6	264
Nonidentical twins			
Men	12.3	5.5	733
Women	14.5	5.7	653

case of the important statistical idea of using homogeneous "blocks" to test
different effects.   First, keeping close to the twin idea, in agricultural experiments, littermates are sometimes assigned to different treatments such as feed-
ing regimes to improve the precision of the resulting average weight gains
under the different diets.   Of course, many litters may need to be used, but
fewer individuals will be needed because of the "matching" provided by the
litters.

Future International Collaboration.   The results from the Scandinavian Twin
Registries show how useful such data can be.   Unfortunately, for less common
diseases even large national registries may not uncover enough cases of a specific
disease (as in different forms of heart disorder) to make detailed statistical
analysis possible.   The World Health Organization therefore has set up a
"registry of registries" to collect data in a uniform fashion in many countries
and assemble and analyze them centrally.   In this way, we hope to reap
the full benefit of the unique research opportunities that studies of twins
in sickness and health can provide.

PROBLEMS

1.   Why are volunteer series in twin studies likely to be biased? (Hint:
refer to the essay by Meier.)

2.   By comparing the risk of an identical twin being affected to that of
a non-identical twin, an experimenter would eliminate any _____
factors, and thus any observed differences between the two kinds of
twins could be attributed to _____ factors.

3. In the data of Table 3, only those pairs of twins are considered for which:
   a. Either both are smokers or nonsmokers.
   b. One twin is a smoker and the other a nonsmoker.
   c. Either both or one or none are smokers.

Which answer is correct?

4. Refer to Table 3. Can you convert the data of cough prevalence from percentage into incidence (number of cases)? Carry out this conversion for the "Identical twins" if you can; explain what other information you need, if you can't.

5. Explain how one should use twins in studies to detect:
   a. The effect of genetic factors in disease.
   b. The effect of environmental factors in disease.

REFERENCES

M. G. Bulmer. 1970. *The Biology of Twinning in Man.* New York: Oxford University Press.

A fuller account of "The Use of Twins in Epidemiological Studies" is given in a WHO report in *Acta Genetica et Gemellologia,* 15(1966):2, pp. 109–128. The Danish Registry and its work are described in the same journal, 18(1968):2, pp. 315–330. The report "Multiple Births USA 1964" from the National Center for Health Statistics is published by the U.S. Public Health Service.

ACKNOWLEDGMENTS

The American Association for the Advancement of Science for permission to publish the figure on p. 16, from Raymond Pearl (1938), "Tobacco Smoking and Longevity," *Science,*87: March 4, pp. 216–217.

American Journal of Public Health for permission to publish the table on p. 97, adapted from T. Francis et al. (1955), "An Evaluation of the 1954 Poliomyelitis Vaccine Trials—Summary Report," *American Journal of Public Health,* 45:5 (Part 2), pp. 1–63.

Atlantic Monthly and David D. Rutstein for permission to publish the figure on p. 92, from D. D. Rutstein (1957), "How Good is Polio Vaccine?" *Atlantic Monthly,* 199:48. Copyright © 1957 Atlantic Monthly Co., Boston, Mass.

Oxford University Press for permission to adapt "How Frequently Do Innovations Succeed in Surgery and Anesthesia?", pp. 51–64, from Bunker, Barnes, and Mosteller (eds.), *Costs, Risks, and Benefits of Surgery,* 1977.

Royal Statistical Society for permission to publish the tables on pp. 8 and 10, from M. S. Bartlett (1957), "Measles Periodicity and Community Size," *Journal of the Royal Statistical Society-A,* 120, pp. 48–70.

INDEX

Adams, John Quincy, 122, 124
Adams, Samuel, 123
Adjustment of rates, 103, 107
Affected concordance rate, 128
Age analysis, 27
Age distribution, 77
Agricultural experiment, 14
Alcohol, 33
Allen, K. R., 30
American Cancer Society, 12, 18
American Museum of Natural History, 70
Analgesics, 32, 33
Analysis of variance, 58, 59
Anesthesia, 51–64
Anesthetics, 101–109
Antarctic, 24
Anthropology, 65–74
Antibody, 90
Ape-or-human example, 65–74
Arnow, L. E., 30, 31
Aureomycin, 30
Australopethecines, 66
Average, 67

Baby boom, 76
Baleen plates, 24
Barnes, B. A., 64
Bartlett, Maurice S., 1–11
Bell, Alexander Graham, 122
Berkson, Joseph, 19, 22
Bias, 15, 17, 20, 95
Bioassay, 20, 32–38, 39–50
Biographies, 122
Biologists, 67
Birth control, 82
Birthday, 111–125
Birth rates, 75–87
Blocking, 132
Blue whales, 25
Blum, J. J., 37
Bronchial asthma, 129
Bronchitis, 131
Brower, Lincoln P., 37
Brown, B. W., Jr., 12–23

Brownlee, K. Alexander, 100
Bulmer, M. G., 133
Bunker, John P., 64, 110

Cancer, 12, 40
Catch-per-day method, 27
Causation, 17
Census, 75
Cerebral apoplexy, 129
Chapman, D. G., 24–31
Children, 122
Chimpanzee, 66
Cigarettes, 13
Cochran, William G., 21
Cocktail party, 32
Columbus, Christopher, 13
Common culture, 122
Community, critical size of, 2, 8
Computer, 66, 77
Concordance, 128
Conservation, 24–31
Control group, 15, 41, 93, 131
Controlled trials, 52
Coppinger, Lorna L., 38
Coronary occlusion, 129
Counterpredictions, 84
Counting methods, 26
Crease, R., 38
Critical threshold, 4
Cumulative distribution, 58
Curare, 34
Cyclopropane, 103

Danish Twin Registry, 128
Davis, Jefferson, 122
Day of Atonement, 124
Deathday, 111–125
Death dip, 113
Death rates, 18, 28, 63, 75–87, 102, 107, 111–125
Death rise, 115
Decision problem, 41
Decision theory, 22
Demographic transition, 305
Demography, 75–87